PRACTICAL
Carbohydrate
Counting 2nd Edition
A How-to-Teach Guide for Health Professionals

Hope S. Warshaw, MMSc, RD, CDE, BC-ADM, and
Karen M. Bolderman, RD, LDN, CDE

American Diabetes Association

Cure • Care • Commitment®

Director, Book Publishing, Robert Anthony; *Managing Editor, Book Publishing,* Abe Ogden; *Acquisitions Editor, Professional Books,* Victor Van Beuren; *Production Manager,* Melissa Sprott; *Composition,* American Diabetes Association; *Cover Design,* Koncept, Inc.; *Printer,* Worzalla Publishing.

Printed in the United States of America
3 5 7 9 10 8 6 4

The suggestions and information contained in this publication are generally consistent with the *Clinical Practice Recommendations* and other policies of the American Diabetes Association, but they do not represent the policy or position of the Association or any of its boards or committees. Reasonable steps have been taken to ensure the accuracy of the information presented. However, the American Diabetes Association cannot ensure the safety or efficacy of any product or service described in this publication. Individuals are advised to consult a physician or other appropriate health care professional before undertaking any diet or exercise program or taking any medication referred to in this publication. Professionals must use and apply their own professional judgment, experience, and training and should not rely solely on the information contained in this publication before prescribing any diet, exercise, or medication. The American Diabetes Association—its officers, directors, employees, volunteers, and members—assumes no responsibility or liability for personal or other injury, loss, or damage that may result from the suggestions or information in this publication.

⊚ The paper in this publication meets the requirements of the ANSI Standard Z39.48-1992 (permanence of paper).

ADA titles may be purchased for business or promotional use or for special sales. To purchase more than 50 copies of this book at a discount, or for custom editions of this book with your logo, contact Lee Romano Sequeira, Special Sales & Promotions, at the address below, or at LRomano@diabetes.org or 703-299-2046.

For all other inquiries, please call 1-800-DIABETES.

American Diabetes Association
1701 North Beauregard Street
Alexandria, Virginia 22311

Library of Congress Cataloging-in-Publication Data

Warshaw, Hope S., 1954-
    Practical carbohydrate counting : a how-to-teach guide for health professionals / by Hope S. Warshaw, Karen M. Bolderman. -- 2nd ed.
        p. ; cm.
    Includes bibliographical references and index.
    ISBN 978-1-58040-282-8 (alk. paper)
    1. Diabetics--Nutrition--Study and teaching. 2. Diabetes--Diet therapy--Study and teaching. 3. Food--Carbohydrate content--Study and teaching. 4. Patient education. I. Bolderman, Karen M., 1954- II. American Diabetes Association. III. Title.
    [DNLM: 1. Diabetes Mellitus--diet therapy. 2. Diabetic Diet--methods. 3. Dietary Carbohydrates--analysis. 4. Patient Education as Topic. WK 818 W295p 2008]

RC662.W3153 2008
616.4'620654071--dc22
                                            2008020554

Table of Contents

Appendices

Introduction

According to the American Diabetes Association (ADA), Medical Nutrition Therapy (MNT) is an integral component of diabetes management and diabetes self-management training (DSMT) (ADA 2008b). MNT has been shown, through clinical trials and outcome studies, to demonstrate decreases in A1C of approximately 1% in type 1 diabetes and 1–2% in type 2 diabetes (Pastors et al. 2002; Pastors, Franz, et al. 2003). By helping patients choose foods and plan meals to monitor their carbohydrate intake and achieve their MNT and diabetes care goals, carbohydrate counting is an attractive meal-planning approach (ADA 2008b).

The following MNT goals for diabetes management (ADA 2008b) are to:

1. Achieve and maintain (refer to Table I-1 for these goals):
   a. Blood glucose levels in the normal range or as close to normal as is safely possible.
   b. A lipid and lipoprotein profile that reduces the risk for vascular disease.
   c. Blood pressure levels in the normal range or as close to normal as is safely possible.

2. Prevent, or at least slow, the rate of development of the chronic complications of diabetes by modifying nutrient intake and lifestyle.

3. Address individual nutrition needs, taking into account personal and cultural preferences and willingness to change.

4. Maintain the pleasure of eating by limiting food choices only when indicated by scientific evidence.

Table I-1. Target Glycemic Goals for Adults with Diabetes

A1C	<7.0%*
Preprandial capillary plasma glucose	70–130 mg/dl (3.9–7.2 mmol/l)
Peak postprandial capillary plasma glucose†	<180 mg/dl (<10.0 mmol/l)

Key concepts in setting glycemic goals:
- A1C is the primary target for glycemic control
- Goals should be individualized based on:
  - duration of diabetes
  - pregnancy status
  - age
  - comorbid conditions
  - hypoglycemia unawareness
  - individual patient considerations
- More stringent glycemic goals (i.e., a normal A1C, <6%) may further reduce complications at the cost of increased risk of hypoglycemia
- Postprancial glucose may be targeted if A1C goals are not met despite reaching preprandial glucose goals.

*Referenced to a nondiabetic range of 4.0–6.0% using a DCCT-based assay.
†Postprandial glucose measurements should be made 1–2 h after the beginning of the meal, generally peak levels in patients with diabetes.
Source: Reprinted by permission from *American Diabetes Association: Clinical Practice Recommendations 2008* (American Diabetes Association, 2008), S18, table 8

Regarding glycemic goals for infants, children, and adolescents, the ADA position statement *Care of Children and Adolescents with Type 1 Diabetes* states that near-normalization of blood glucose levels in children and adolescents is generally the same as that for adults (ADA 2005). However, the position statement details a number of caveats that discuss the greater risks of hypoglycemia and the difficulty of achieving tight glycemic control in this age population. The position statement specifies A1C goals that differ from the adult A1C goal for three age groups as follows:

- Children <6 years old: 7.5–8.5%
- Children 6–12 years old: < 8%
- Adolescents: 7.5%

Making the necessary lifestyle changes to eat healthy with diabetes, in addition to acquiring and utilizing the knowledge to both prospectively and retrospectively manage glycemic control acutely and chronically, is one of the most challenging aspects of diabetes care. Helping people with diabetes achieve these goals is also challenging for their providers. Many factors contribute to the challenge of glycemic control, including those listed in Table I-2. Yet, it has been shown that people at varying levels of ability and motivation, as well as people implementing various diabetes therapies, can use carbohydrate counting to achieve short- and long-term glycemic and health goals (Anderson et al. 1993; DAFNE Study Group 2002).

Table I-2. Interrelated Factors That Determine Plasma Glucose Concentration

Numerous interrelated factors determine plasma glucose concentration in people with diabetes*, including:

1. Carbohydrate composition of food
2. Rate of gastric emptying
3. Rate of glucose absorption
4. Concurrent magnitude of endogenous glucose production
5. Concurrent rate of glucose disposal
6. Diurnal change in insulin sensitivity
7. Activity of counterregulatory hormones
8. Change in the magnitude and type of exercise
9. Ambient insulin concentration
10. Consumption of alcohol
11. Acute illness
12. Emotional stress

*This list constitutes a lengthy, yet incomplete, list of interrelated factors that affect plasma glucose. Several were listed in reference (Schade and Valentine 2006).

To help facilitate these established health outcomes, *Practical Carbohydrate Counting: A How-to-Teach Guide for Health Professionals* is designed to:

1. Provide educators with the concepts to cover when teaching Basic and Advanced Carbohydrate Counting

2. Help educators learn how to assess preexisting knowledge and abilities and determine if and when a person is ready to progress their level of carbohydrate counting

3. Discuss related dietary and nondietary factors, beyond the carbohydrate content of foods, that affect blood glucose control

4. Utilize case studies for Basic and Advanced Carbohydrate Counting that illustrate the use of this meal planning approach

5. Offer educators a variety of carbohydrate counting resources

CHAPTER ONE

What, Why, Who, and How Much?

CARBOHYDRATE COUNTING DEFINED

Carbohydrate Counting is an approach to meal planning that is often considered as two distinct methods with appropriate goals for each: Basic Carbohydrate Counting, a simpler approach, and Advanced Carbohydrate Counting, a progression of skills that entail more complex and time-intensive teaching. However, Basic and Advanced Carbohydrate Counting can also be considered a continuum of a single meal-planning approach, since a person must first master the concepts and skills of Basic Carbohydrate Counting before he or she can progress to Advanced Carbohydrate Counting.

The goals of Basic Carbohydrate Counting are, as expected, relatively minimal and often limited to learning the foods that contain carbohydrate and demonstrating knowledge of how to choose and eat these foods in the proper portions. People using Basic Carbohydrate Counting are encouraged to eat consistent amounts of carbohydrate at meals and snacks at similar times each day, with the end goal of achieving glycemic control and other diabetes and metabolic nutrition goals. Basic Carbohydrate Counting is most appropriate for people with type 2 diabetes who control their diabetes with a healthy eating plan and physical activity, with or without the addition of one or more blood glucose–lowering medications.

The individual goals of Advanced Carbohydrate Counting are more varied and complex, but designed with the overarching objective of helping a person learn to synchronize the amount of glucose-lowering medication they take with the amount of carbohydrate consumed. This method of carbohydrate counting works well with the use of multiple blood glucose–lowering medications (see Appendix II), including oral agents and injectable medications, but is especially suited to multiple daily injection (MDI) insulin regimens or a continuous sub-cutaneous insulin infusion pump (CSII), commonly known as insulin pump therapy.

People using Advanced Carbohydrate Counting are taught to use customized insulin-to-carbohydrate ratios (ICR) that are calculated based on their individual insulin and carbohydrate needs. They are also taught how to use a customized correction factor (CF), sometimes referred to as insulin sensitivity factor, to correct hyperglycemia and/or prevent further or future hypoglycemia. Ultimately, the use of Advanced Carbohydrate Counting is intended to help people enjoy a more flexible food and medication regimen that is more suited to contemporary daily life while simultaneously achieving improved glycemic control.

Both the Basic and Advanced methods of Carbohydrate Counting are fully described in later chapters.

THE CASE FOR CARBOHYDRATE COUNTING

Carbohydrate counting has grown in popularity as a meal planning approach in the United States since the completion of the Diabetes Complications and Control Trial (DCCT), in which carbohydrate counting was effectively used (Anderson et al. 1993; DCCT 1993). However, carbohydrate counting has been in use internationally since insulin was discovered and has been the meal planning method of choice in the United Kingdom for years (McCulloch et al. 1993).

Carbohydrate Counting has become popular for several reasons. First, the priority of achieving and maintaining glycemic control to decrease morbidity and mortality from diabetes complications has gained greater importance due to the results of the DCCT (DCCT 1993) and the United Kingdom Prospective Diabetes Study (UKPDS) in people with type 2 diabetes (UKPDS 1998). According to the American Diabetes Association's (ADA) most recent nutrition recommendations and interventions, control of blood glucose to achieve glycemic control is a primary goal of diabetes management (ADA 2008b). Second, more attention is now focused on postprandial blood glucose control (Parkin and Brooks 2002) because of the finding that it is more strongly associated with the risks for atherosclerosis than preprandial blood glucose (Temelkova-Kurktschiev 2000). People with diabetes have defects in insulin action, insulin secretion, or both, and insulin defects impair the regulation of postprandial glucose in response to carbohydrate intake. The quantity and the type/source of carbohydrate intake are the major determinants of postprandial glucose levels (ADA 2008b). Interventions to help people accurately count and control their carbohydrate intake are important to help improve postprandial glycemic control.

The ADA suggests that carbohydrate counting is one method of meal planning that can help people match their doses of some blood glucose–lowering medications, such as insulin and/or insulin secretagogues, to carbohydrate consumption (ADA 2008b). Further, the Dose Adjusted for Normal Eating (DAFNE) trial conducted in Great Britain demonstrated a 1% lowering of A1C in people with type 1 diabetes who received training in adjusting mealtime insulin based on the carbohydrate consumed (DAFNE Study Group 2002).

RECOMMENDATIONS FOR CARBOHYDRATE CONSUMPTION

Total carbohydrate

The following is a brief review of the current ADA recommendations regarding the consumption of carbohydrate within the framework of a healthy eating plan (ADA 2008b). More extensive reviews can be found (ADA 2008b; Sheard et al. 2004). Regarding the percent of calories that carbohydrate should contribute to the mix of macronutrients, the ADA states that "it is unlikely that one such combination of macronutrients exists that is optimal for all people with diabetes" (ADA 2008b). The ADA recommendations suggest that people seek guidance from the Institute of Medicine's *Dietary Reference Intakes* (DRIs) (Institute of Medicine 2002). The DRIs recommend that adults should consume 45–65% of total energy from carbohydrate to meet the body's daily nutritional needs while minimizing risk for chronic diseases.

The ADA supports the use of either low-carbohydrate or low-fat calorie-restricted diets for short-term use in people with diabetes. For longer term use, the ADA continues to raise questions about the long-term metabolic effects of very low–carbohydrate diets, which eliminate many foods that are important sources of energy, fiber, and other essential nutrients (ADA 2008b). The DRIs indicate that the minimum adult requirement for carbohydrate to provide adequate glucose for the central nervous system without reliance on protein or fat is 130 grams per day (Institute of Medicine 2002; Sheard et al. 2004). The ADA recommends, as do the DRIs, that good health can be achieved with a pattern of food intake that includes carbohydrate from fruits, vegetables, whole grains, legumes, and low-fat milk (ADA 2008b; Institute of Medicine 2002). It is worth noting that contemporary patterns of food intake are often lacking in foods from these groups (U.S. Department of Health and Human Services 2005). The remainder of calories can be contributed by 20–35% from fat and 10–35% from protein (Institute of Medicine 2002).

Amounts and types of carbohydrate

As noted above, the ADA nutrition recommendations suggest that carbohydrate intake, both the quantity and the type or source of carbohydrate, is the major determinant of postprandial glucose levels (ADA 2008b). With this stated, it should be noted that the ADA recommendations now reflect that the use of the Glycemic Index (GI) and Glycemic Load (GL) as a means to assess the glycemic impact of a food on blood glucose can provide a modest additional benefit over that observed when just total carbohydrate is considered (ADA 2008b). The concepts of GI and GL are discussed further in chapter 10, along with other dietary components that impact blood glucose levels, including fiber, polyols, protein, and fat.

Basic Carbohydrate Counting

CHAPTER TWO

Assessing Knowledge and Skills

The choice to use carbohydrate counting as a meal planning approach should be based on several factors about each individual, including but not limited to

- Existing knowledge of meal planning and diabetes management self-management
- Willingness and ability to learn and use the necessary skills
- Diabetes management needs and desires

These same factors will indicate whether a person should progress from Basic to Advanced Carbohydrate Counting (see chapter 6).

ASSESSING A PERSON'S KNOWLEDGE AND SKILLS

Before beginning carbohydrate counting education, it is essential to determine a person's base knowledge. When working with a person with newly diagnosed diabetes or new to carbohydrate counting, assess the following:

- Knowledge of the goals for healthy eating in general
- Knowledge of the goals for healthy eating with diabetes
- Preconceived notions of what a person with diabetes should or should not eat, as well as understanding about the timing of meals and snacks
- Understanding of basic nutrition concepts, such as:
  - The three macronutrients—carbohydrate, protein, and fat
  - Foods that provide the three main macronutrients
- Understanding of blood glucose–lowering medication(s)—onset, action, duration, and mechanism(s) of action(s)

People with diabetes are referred for medical nutrition therapy (MNT) at varying points in their life and management of diabetes. For this reason, it is important to realize that just because a person has had diabetes for many years or claims to have learned or used carbohydrate counting, doesn't mean that they have and/or are able to apply the above knowledge and/or that this knowledge is up to date as diabetes nutrition recommendations have evolved.

Methods for assessment

Since many diabetes educators teach Basic Carbohydrate Counting in a group setting, it is important to develop methods that assess each person's knowledge and learning needs within the group. Consider using one or more of these assessment options:

- Develop a few written questions that allow you to quickly assess whether people know the foods (as food groups) that do and do not contain carbohydrate (see box Questions to Ask).
- Ask people to complete a one-to-three day food record and have them circle the foods that contain carbohydrate. Ask them to include the amount of food and, if possible, the amount of carbohydrate each food provides. If people haven't determined the carbohydrate counts

Questions to Ask

Below are some questions educators may want to pose to assess a person's existing knowledge and use of carbohydrate counting:

- What are the foods/food groups that contain sources of carbohydrate?
- What are the foods/food groups that contain no carbohydrate?
- What is the impact of various foods (macronutrients) on blood glucose?

In addition, educators should ask people who state that they use Advanced Carbohydrate Counting these key questions:

- Do you have an insulin-to-carbohydrate ratio (ICR)?
- Do you have a correction factor (CF)?
- If so, how do you go about using these to calculate your rapid-acting insulin doses?

Information about a person's existing knowledge, preconceived notions, and previous education help the educator determine the individual's base knowledge and learning needs.

of these foods, they can demonstrate their ability to do this using a variety of carbohydrate counting resources and tools provided by the educator in class (see box Tools and Resources Every Educator Needs). Finally, have them provide a total carbohydrate count for meals and for the day.

- To assess a person's measuring skills, consider having a box of dry cereal, nuts, or dried fruit (foods that can be reused and aren't perishable), and ask them to measure out a specific amount or one serving of the food.
- Provide people with different Nutrition Facts panels from common packaged foods. Create a brief questionnaire that can demonstrate their knowledge of where to find the serving size and total grams of carbohydrate. Determine if they can calculate the total grams in a serving if the serving is different from the serving size on the Nutrition Facts panel.
- Use food models to ask people to estimate the carbohydrate count of a variety of foods, including commonly eaten mixed dishes.
- Develop a brief questionnaire with which to assess a person's ability to find and determine a total for the grams of carbohydrate in a fast food meal. Use the nutrition facts for fast food restaurants (see Appendix I).

Ongoing assessment

In addition to assessing initial carbohydrate counting skills, it is important to be able to assess the progression of a person's knowledge and skills as well.

Tools and Resources Every Educator Needs

The following list of visual aids, reading materials, and other equipment can make assessing skills and teaching carbohydrate counting easier and more effective.

- Nutrition Facts panels from food labels
- Measuring equipment
- Nonperishable, reusable food products that people can measure
- Resources that list carbohydrate counts of foods—from basic foods to restaurant foods (for which nutrition information is available)
- Restaurant menus and nutrition facts for the menu items
- Calculator
- Food models or pictures of foods from which people can divide foods into those that contain carbohydrate and those that do not

Educators can use many of the same questions and tools suggested above for this purpose.

Assessment Checklist

Below is a list of knowledge and skills a person using Basic Carbohydrate Counting should obtain. Some of the skills may be present from the beginning; most will probably be acquired through carbohydrate counting education. Use this checklist as an ongoing assessment tool. Strategies for teaching this knowledge and these skills are addressed in chapters 3 and 4.

Covered in *Chapter 3. Concepts to Teach—From Basic Nutrition to Meal Planning*:

☐ Understand the rationale behind why carbohydrate counting can effectively achieve glycemic control
☐ Identify the foods (food groups) that contain carbohydrate
☐ Identify the foods (food groups) that do not contain carbohydrate
☐ Understand that foods that contain carbohydrate are healthy and offer energy and an array of vitamins and minerals
☐ Understand that healthy foods that contain carbohydrate should not be significantly limited or avoided as a means to achieve glycemic control (if a person is not achieving glycemic goals, other methods, such as blood glucose–lowering medication, should be utilized, constituting a progression of therapy)
☐ Know how much carbohydrate to eat per day
☐ Know how much carbohydrate to eat at meals and snacks
☐ Define a serving of a variety of common foods
☐ Know how to plan meals
☐ Know how to integrate limited amounts of sucrose-containing foods into a healthy eating plan
☐ Have general personal guidelines for what and how much protein and fat to eat
☐ Know how to take, record, and track blood glucose levels

Covered in *Chapter 4. Concepts to Teach—Counting Carb, Reading Food Labels, and Measuring Portions*:

☐ Know how to determine the carbohydrate counts of foods
☐ Know how to use the Nutrition Facts panel
☐ Have and know how to use measuring equipment and portion control tools and tips
☐ Know how to interpret postprandial blood glucose levels

Progression to Advanced Carbohydrate Counting

A person who is ready to progress to learning and using Advanced Carbo-hydrate Counting should be able to perform all the tasks listed above in the Assessment Checklist. However, not all diabetes self-management regimens are suited to Advanced Carbohydrate Counting. The mastery of Basic Carbohydrate Counting—with the simple goal of eating a consistent amount of carbohydrate throughout the day—can be an endpoint for some people with diabetes. For others, the mastery of Basic Carbohydrate Counting skills and knowledge will serve as a base upon which they can progress to acquire and master Advanced Carbohydrate Counting skills.

A person who has type 2 diabetes and follows a healthy eating plan inte-grated with regular physical activity and no blood glucose–lowering medications has no need to progress to Advanced Carbohydrate Counting with their current regimen. They may need to progress as their diabetes management plan becomes more complex, often with the addition of oral or injectable medications and/or insulin that can be adjusted based on blood glucose levels and/or carbohydrate intake. Until that time (or if that complexity never becomes necessary), Basic Carbohydrate Counting will usually suffice.

In other cases, there is no intermediary period between Basic and Advanced Carbohydrate Counting. The person with type 1 diabetes who seeks a more flex-ible insulin regimen and eating plan may want or need to progress beyond Basic Carbohydrate Counting immediately. Chapter 6 provides a more in-depth dis-cussion of determining a person's readiness to progress.

CHAPTER THREE

Concepts to Teach— From Basic Nutrition to Meal Planning

Regardless of the initial knowledge level or ultimate goals of the person learning carbohydrate counting as a meal planning approach, all will begin with Basic Carbohydrate Counting. In chapter 2 we discussed assessing carbohydrate counting skills and presented an Assessment Checklist (see page 14) that summarized the necessary skills involved with Basic Carbohydrate Counting. In this chapter, we'll discuss many of those concepts and some strategies for teaching those concepts.

CONCEPTS TO TEACH

Rationale for counting carbohydrate

It is important that a person understands the rationale for counting carbohydrate. Give a brief explanation that calories are provided from three macronutrients—carbohydrate, protein, and fat. Next explain that foods are made up of combinations, or "packages" of varying amounts of carbohydrate, protein, and fat.

Concrete examples work best, so provide examples in terms of real foods. The following examples often work well:

- A slice of bread (white or whole wheat) contains mainly carbohydrate and a small amount of protein.
- A piece of grilled chicken contains mainly protein and a small amount of fat.
- A piece of fruit contains mainly carbohydrate.
- A glass of milk (8 ounces) contains mainly carbohydrate, but is also a source of protein and may contain some fat, depending on the type of milk.

After you've established carbohydrate as a constituent of food and given some general examples of carbohydrate-containing foods, move on to the role carbohydrate plays in diabetes self-management. Some concepts to explain:

- It is the carbohydrate in foods that is the main contributor to the rise of blood glucose after eating. Carbohydrate counting as a meal planning approach focuses on counting the amount of the nutrient (carbohydrate) that causes the greatest rise in blood glucose levels.
- Equivalent amounts of carbohydrate from a variety of carbohydrate-containing foods raise blood glucose to about the same degree in about the same amount of time (ADA 2008b).
- There are some foods and some factors about the qualities of food that may cause them to raise blood glucose faster or slower than others.
- To help keep blood glucose in control while following a healthy meal plan, it's important to consume healthy sources of carbohydrate in consistent amounts through the day.
- When foods that provide mainly protein (meat, fish, etc.) and fat are eaten in amounts consistent with a healthy eating plan, they raise blood glucose levels minimally.

Identify foods (food groups) that contain carbohydrate

Ensure that the person knows the list of foods (food groups) that contain carbohydrate. Do not assume that people know this. It is quite common for people to equate starches with carbohydrate and have no knowledge that foods such as fruits, milk, and ice cream also contain carbohydrate.

Food groups that contain carbohydrate:

- Starches, including breads, grains, and cereals
- Starchy vegetables, including beans (legumes)
- Fruit and fruit juices
- Vegetables (nonstarchy)
- Milk, yogurt, ice cream, and some other dairy foods
- Sugary foods
- Sweets and desserts
- Fat-free foods (often in the form of carbohydrate-based fat replacers)
- Sugar-free foods (which contain polyols)

Identify foods (food groups) that do not contain carbohydrate

Assure that the person also knows the list of foods (food groups) that do not contain carbohydrate.

Food groups that do not contain carbohydrate:

- Meats, seafood, poultry
- Eggs
- Cheese (hard and soft cheeses contain minimal carbohydrate)
- Fats, such as margarine, butter, and mayonnaise (Note: Do point out that some fats, such as commercially prepared salad dressings, do contain some carbohydrate. Also point out that many fat-free foods contain some carbohydrate.)
- Oils
- Nuts (other than chestnuts, which contain minimal carbohydrate)

Understand that many foods that contain carbohydrate are healthy and offer energy and an array of vitamins and minerals

A common reaction, once a person realizes that carbohydrate raises blood glucose levels, is to eat less carbohydrate than is recommended for health and healthy eating. This belief is also cultivated by promises of low-carbohydrate, high-protein diets to improve metabolic control and produce weight loss. People often don't know that sources of carbohydrate are not the same and carbohydrate-containing foods essentially fall into two groups—healthier and less healthy sources of carbohydrate. People also often think that the current American diet is high in total carbohydrate, which is untrue. Americans eat about 50 percent of their calories as carbohydrate. The concern is that a large percent of carbohydrate intake is from added sugars, as opposed to more desirable sources (U.S. Department of Health and Human Services et al. 2005).

Consider teaching the following points:

- Many carbohydrate-containing foods are among the healthiest foods to eat: whole grains, fruits, vegetables, and low- or fat-free milk and yogurt (Institute of Medicine 2002). Carbohydrate-containing foods are the body's primary and preferred sources of energy and provide many essential vitamins and minerals. Also, whole grains and many fruits, vegetables, and starchy vegetables are the body's main source of various types of dietary fiber.
- Delineate between healthier food sources of carbohydrate and less healthy sources. Today, Americans in general eat insufficient amounts of healthy carbohydrates and overconsume less healthy carbohydrates (U.S. Department of Health and Human Services et al. 2005).
  Less than healthy sources to mention:
  - Sugary foods

- Regular sodas
- Fruit drinks and other calorie-rich, sweetened beverages
- Sweets and desserts
- Refined snack foods

- Reinforce that careful attention to the portion size of carbohydrate-containing foods is critical to achieving blood glucose control—even when eating healthier sources of carbohydrate.
- Many people ask when they need to start counting carbohydrate from nonstarchy vegetables. This question is often beside the point, since most people do not consume enough nonstarchy vegetables. For most, the amount of carbohydrate from nonstarchy vegetables at meals is likely <10 grams of carbohydrate. However, people who eat several servings (about 1 cup raw, 1/2 cup cooked) of vegetables at meals should count the carbohydrate once it equals 10 grams or more. Educators should certainly encourage people to eat more nonstarchy vegetables, but also note that large quantities of some vegetables, such as carrots and tomatoes, can affect blood glucose.

Understand that healthy foods that contain carbohydrate should not be significantly limited or avoided as a means to achieve glycemic control

Reinforce the message that blood glucose control should not be achieved by avoiding healthy foods. Limiting foods that contain healthy sources of carbohydrate can compromise nutritional status.

Some people with type 2 diabetes facing the need to start an oral or injectable blood glucose–lowering medication may attempt to limit carbohydrate intake as a means to lower blood glucose. They believe that this will further delay the need to add or transition to new medication regimens. For this reason, it is important to discuss with them the common progression of type 2 diabetes. People need to understand that, as time goes on, they will produce less insulin and continue to have insulin resistance. They will need to introduce and/or modify their blood glucose–lowering medication to continue to achieve target blood glucose goals.

Know how much carbohydrate to eat per day

A person's need for carbohydrate relates to his or her calorie needs. Calorie and carbohydrate needs depend on numerous factors:

- Height
- Weight and weight history

- Usual food habits and daily schedule
- Level of physical activity
- Blood glucose control
- Blood lipid levels

The current American Diabetes Association (ADA) nutrition recommendations note that no optimal nutrient mix for carbohydrate, protein, and fat has been determined for people with diabetes (ADA 2008b) and that the *Dietary Reference Intake* (DRI) of 45–65% of total calories from carbohydrate is reasonable to follow (Institute of Medicine 2002). On average, Americans eat about 50% of their calories as carbohydrate, although a greater than desirable percent of these calories comes from less healthy carbohydrate sources (Institute of Medicine 2002; U.S. Department of Health and Human Services et al. 2005). It is optimal to individualize carbohydrate intake based on the above factors and healthy eating goals. Table 3-1 provides general guidelines for the amount of total daily carbohydrate intake and servings from food groups for various calorie ranges. As provided, these would supply approximately 50% of calories as carbohydrate, 20% as protein, and 30% as fat.

Know how much carbohydrate to eat at meals and snacks

The number of meals and snacks a person eats should be based on two factors: current food habits and daily schedule. Understanding a person's food habits and general daily schedule casts light on blood glucose results and control. Find out if the person is a three-meal-a-day eater, a person who finds it helpful to snack between meals, or a three-meal-a day eater and nighttime snacker. Learn about how and why a person divides his or her food between the number of meals and snacks he or she eats each day. Perhaps the person barely eats breakfast and eats a large evening meal. This might be why blood glucose levels after the evening meal are higher than at other times of the day. If the person eats snacks, find out why.

In addition, review the types and doses of blood glucose–lowering medications he or she has been prescribed. Overlay this information with their food intake and daily schedule. Then think about how well this routine works for them or whether a change in his or her medication and/or medication schedule may improve glycemic control. Keep in mind that it is easier for someone to change a medication or medication regimen than to change lifelong food habits.

After exploring and considering the above factors, divide the total amount of carbohydrate into meals and possibly one or more snacks. Strive for a balance of carbohydrate throughout the day and a similar amount of carbohydrate at meals and snacks from day to day. However, keep the person's food habits in mind.

Table 3-1. Daily Carbohydrate Needs

Physical profile, activity level and nutrition goals	Women (small stature and/or older) who desire weight loss, are small in stature and/or sedentary	Women (small stature, older, and/or sedentary) who desire weight maintenance or larger women who desire weight loss
Calorie Range[1]	1200 – 1400	1400 – 1600
Carbohydrate (g)[2] (~50% of calories)	160	180
Carbohydrate (servings/day, serving equals 15 g of carb)[3]	10	11
Servings per day:		
Grains, beans, and starchy vegetables[2]	5	6
Fruits	3	3
Milk[3]	2	2
Vegetables (nonstarchy)	3	4
Meats[4]	5 oz	6 oz
Grams[5]	45	55
Servings (serving equals 5 g fat)[6]	5	6

Notes:
1. The groups of people for whom these calorie ranges are appropriate generalizations.
2. The total grams of carbohydrate and servings of carbohydrate are from grains, beans, and starchy vegetables; fruits; and milk. Nonstarchy vegetables are not counted in the amount for carbohydrate servings, but are counted in the total grams of carbohydrate.
3. Based on fat-free milk (12 grams of carbohydrate and 8 grams of protein per 8 ounces). Children between 9 and 18 years old need 1300 milligrams of calcium per day. They should get at least three servings per day of milk. Adults from 19 to 50 need 1000 milligrams of calcium per day. This can be met with two servings of milk a day, plus another serving of a high-calcium food. Women over

Women (moderate to large stature) who are active and desire weight maintenance. Older men, and men (small to moderate stature) who desire weight loss	Children, teen girls, and active larger women, men (small to moderate stature) who desire weight maintenance. Men (large stature and active) who desire weight loss	Teen boys, active teen girls and active men (moderate to large stature) who desire weight maintenance
1600 – 1900	1900 – 2300	2300 – 2800
210	260	305
13	16	19
8	10	12
3	4	5
2	2	2
4	5	5
6 oz	7 oz	8 oz
60	75	90
8	10	13

51 years of age need 1200 milligrams of calcium per day. If milk or another excellent source of dairy is not regularly consumed, suggest the use of a calcium supplement to achieve the daily calcium goal. Then suggest adding another 24 grams of carbohydrate from either grains, beans, and starchy vegetables or fruit.

4. Calculated based on lean meat figures (7 grams of protein and 3 grams of fat per ounce). Use more or fewer grams or servings of fat based on the type of meats you tend to eat.

5. The calculation for the grams of fat is derived from the fat in meats plus the fat in the fat servings.

6. The servings of fat assume that each serving of fat provides 5 grams of fat.

Recognize that the average American eats a light breakfast, slightly heavier lunch, and the biggest meal at the evening meal.

Note that an eating plan for people with diabetes should no longer automatically include snacks. The rationale in years past for including snacks was to prevent hypoglycemia, a common risk from the then limited array of oral blood glucose–lowering medications and insulins (Polonsky and Jackson 2004). If hypoglycemia is occurring regularly, work with the person to determine the common reasons for their hypoglycemia and develop solutions that involve changes or timing adjustments with blood glucose–lowering medications and/or food intake. Include or eliminate snacks with the goal of achieving a balance between food habits and hypoglycemia prevention (if they take a medication that can cause hypoglycemia). If someone doesn't want to include snacks and is not on blood glucose–lowering medication that can cause hypoglycemia, then snacks are unnecessary. If a person doesn't want to include snacks and is on a multiple daily injection (MDI) insulin regimen or a continuous subcutaneous insulin infusion (CSII) pump, then snacks are unnecessary. An exception comes with young children. If a child has a small appetite at meals or difficult-to-control nighttime hypoglycemia, then snacks (generally three a day) are probably necessary to meet nutrition needs.

Table 3-2 provides a sample handout to help people learn how much carbohydrate to eat, how to divide the carbohydrate into meals and snacks, and space to work out or provide two sample meals.

Define a serving of a variety of common foods

People need to have a sense of how much food represents one, two, or three or more servings of a food that contains carbohydrate. They need to be able to translate the amount of carbohydrate (in either grams or servings) they should eat into real amounts of food. In the language of diabetes exchanges/choices, one serving of a starch, fruit, or milk serving equals about 15 grams of carbohydrate and one serving of nonstarchy vegetables equals about 5 grams of carbohydrate (Pastors, Arnold, et al. 2003). Table 3-3 provides a chart with the average macronutrients per serving in major food groups (Pastors, Arnold, et al. 2003).

The average amounts of carbohydrate in Table 3-3 can be used to teach generalities about the grams of carbohydrate per food group without mentioning the word "exchanges" or "choices." Recognize that as the exchange/choice system is used less frequently to educate people with diabetes (particularly as more educators use carbohydrate counting), fewer people will be familiar with the exchange/choice system. Also recognize that there are different definitions of "servings." Consider the definitions used herein as well as the definitions on the Nutrition Facts panels of foods set by the U.S. FDA. Table 3-4 provides examples of how these can be similar or different.

Table 3-2. How Much Carbohydrate to Eat and When?

Calorie Range: _____ calories/day

Carbohydrate Grams/day: _____

Carbohydrate Servings/day: _____

Breakfast	**Sample Meal**	**Sample Meal**
Time: _____	_____	_____
Carbohydrate Grams ____	_____	_____
Carbohydrate Servings_____	_____	_____

Snack*	**Sample Snack**	**Sample Snack**
Time: _____	_____	_____
Carbohydrate Grams ____	_____	_____
Carbohydrate Servings_____	_____	_____

Lunch	**Sample Meal**	**Sample Meal**
Time: _____	_____	_____
Carbohydrate Grams ____	_____	_____
Carbohydrate Servings_____	_____	_____

Snack*	**Sample Snack**	**Sample Snack**
Time: _____	_____	_____
Carbohydrate Grams ____	_____	_____
Carbohydrate Servings_____	_____	_____

Evening Meal	**Sample Meal**	**Sample Meal**
Time: _____	_____	_____
Carbohydrate Grams ____	_____	_____
Carbohydrate Servings_____	_____	_____

Snack*	**Sample Snack**	**Sample Snack**
Time: _____	_____	_____
Carbohydrate Grams ____	_____	_____
Carbohydrate Servings_____	_____	_____

*Snacks: The inclusion of one, two, or more snacks per day should be dependent on the person's age, nutritional needs, and food habits. People with diabetes, especially when they use newer blood glucose–lowering medications, do not need to include snacks for the purpose of preventing hypoglycemia as was true in the past. It is always best to help people regulate their blood glucose–lowering medication rather than adjusting meal or snack frequency and/or timing.

Table 3-3. Macronutrients per Serving in Major Food Groups

		Nutrients*		
Food Group	Serving†	Carbohydrate (g) 4 calories per gram	Protein (g) 4 calories per gram	Fat (g) 9 calories per gram
Bread	1 slice	15	3	0
Cereal, dry	1 oz	15	3	‡
Cereal, cooked	1/2 cup	15	3	‡
Pasta	1/3 cup	15	3	‡
Starchy vegetable	1/3 to 1/2 cup	15	3	0
Fruit, fresh	1 medium piece	15	0	0
Fruit juice	1/3 to 1/2 cup	15	0	0
Fruit, canned, no sugar added	1/2 cup	15	0	0
Vegetables	1/2 cup cooked	5	0	0
Vegetables	1 cup raw	5	0	0
Milk, fat free	1 cup	12	8	0
Yogurt, plain, nonfat	3/4 cup (6 oz)	12	8	0
Sugary foods	1 serving	Varies	Varies	Varies
Sweets	1 serving	Varies	Varies	Varies
Meats	3 oz cooked	0	21	Varies
Fats—margarine, mayonnaise, oil	1 teaspoon	0	0	5

* Alcohol contains 7 calories per gram and is considered a nutrient.
† Servings are according to servings in *Choose Your Foods: Exchange Lists for Diabetes* (ADA and American Dietetic Association 2007).
‡ Depends on the cereal.

Even as counting grams of carbohydrate grows in popularity, many educators prefer to teach servings of carbohydrate. There is rationale for teaching one or the other or both. Some educators believe that if someone is familiar with the exchange/ choice system and/or the fact that 15 grams of carbohydrate is a serving or one carbohydrate choice, then this knowledge should be used. The downside of only teaching servings (or choices) is that people have no base for translating the Nutrition Facts of food labels or other resources that only provide grams of carbohydrate.

Another downside of teaching exchanges/choices is that it introduces yet another term to a person's carbohydrate counting lexicon. Some educators believe

Table 3-4. Different Sources, Different Serving Sizes

Same (Example)

Food	Diabetes Serving	Food Label Serving
Milk	1 cup/8 ounces	1 cup/8 ounces
Bread	1 slice/1 ounce	1 slice/1 ounce

Different (Example)

Food	Diabetes Serving	Food Label Serving
Fruit juice	1/2 cup/4 ounces	1 cup/8 ounces
Margarine	1 teaspoon regular stick	1 tablespoon regular stick

that teaching people to count grams of carbohydrate is more precise and makes it easier to use the variety of carbohydrate counting resources available. For people learning and using Basic Carbohydrate Counting, providing both a count of carbohydrate grams as well as servings (total and per meal) may be most helpful, as shown in Table 3-2. People who progress to using Advanced Carbohydrate Counting should be trained use the more precise practice of counting grams of carbohydrate. Averaging based on servings will not match medication as precisely.

Know how to plan meals

Converting the recommended servings and grams of carbohydrate into palatable meals is often the most challenging aspect of meal planning for many people with diabetes. People need to have a sense of what and how much they should eat at their meals to gain confidence that this is a plan they can follow. Use a form, such as the one in Table 3-2, to work out two sample meals. In a group setting, this is a form that people can complete and review with an educator. In a one-on-one setting, this is a form that can be completed together. Various teaching tools, such as those in the list on page 13 in chapter 2, can be used to help people gain confidence in this skill. In addition, people may be interested in online meal and menu planning.

Know how to integrate limited amounts of sucrose-containing foods into a healthy eating plan

The current ADA (2008b) nutrition recommendation about the inclusion of sucrose and sucrose-containing foods reads as follows:

> Sucrose-containing foods can be substituted for other carbohydrates in the meal plan or, if added to the meal plan, covered with insulin or other glucose-lowering medications. Care should be taken to avoid excess energy intake.

This recommendation is based on the scientific evidence that dietary sucrose does not increase glycemia more than the same amounts of starch. Sucrose-containing foods do not need to be limited because of a concern about exacerbating hyperglycemia (ADA 2008b). However, it is common for sucrose-containing foods to contain fat, saturated fat, and cholesterol as well as excess calories.

With these recommendations in hand, it is reasonable to teach people with diabetes that sugary foods and sweets have not been forbidden since the publication of the 1994 ADA nutrition recommendations. However, to maintain a healthy eating plan and achieve their diabetes and nutrition goals, sugary foods and sweets usually need to be limited. This recommendation is in sync with the *Dietary Guidelines for Americans* (U.S. Department of Health and Human Services et al. 2005).

In providing individual guidance about sweets, the educator should consider the person's food habits and preferences along with their weight, glycemic, and lipid status. It is reasonable to assume that most people will want to include some sucrose-containing foods in their eating plan and it is important to help them learn how to do this within the context of achieving their nutrition and diabetes goals.

These tips can help people eat fewer and smaller portions of sweets:

- Choose a few favorite desserts and decide how often to eat them based on personal diabetes and nutrition goals.
- Take note of the calories, total fat, saturated fat, and cholesterol of preferred desserts. Make healthier choices.
- Recognize that smaller portions can satisfy the sweet tooth just as much as large portions. For this reason, split desserts when eating out. Take advantage of smaller portions when they are available, such as in ice cream shops, when you can choose the kiddie, junior, single, or regular scoop.
- Use the Nutrition Facts on the food label to learn the grams of carbohydrate per serving. Then use this information to appropriately swap a sucrose-containing food for another carbohydrate-containing food.
- Learn the impact of sucrose-containing foods on blood glucose. Check blood glucose 1 to 2 hours after eating to see the effect. People may find that sucrose-containing foods with more fat raise blood glucose more slowly.
- Explore palatable sugar-free options that are sweetened with no-calorie sweeteners.

Have general guidelines for what and how much protein and fat to eat

As noted, carbohydrate is the main determinant of glycemic rise after eating. Protein and fat have far less impact on the rise of blood glucose levels than carbohydrate (ADA 2008b). Despite the limited impact of protein and fat on blood glucose levels, the amount of these macronutrients consumed by people with diabetes can contribute to both their short- and long-term health. Refer to chapter 10 for more discussion on the impact of protein and fat on blood glucose levels. The ADA encourages practitioners to follow the DRIs for protein of 10–35% of total energy and 20–35% for fat (ADA 2008b; Institute of Medicine 2002).

People who are taught Basic Carbohydrate Counting also need to be provided with some basic guidelines about healthy amounts of foods that contain protein and fat.

Educational points about protein

- Teach the foods (food groups) that provide protein. Teach that foods such as red meats, seafood, eggs, and poultry provide no carbohydrate (unless it is added into a convenience food or in food preparation), but mainly protein and varying amounts of fat. Do note that fat and carbohydrate content of these foods can change based on food preparation. Teach that servings of milk and yogurt provide protein. One cup of milk (any type) provides about the amount of protein as an ounce of meat. Teach that smaller amounts of protein come from non-animal sources, such as grains, cereals, pasta, beans, and vegetables. Use Table 3-3 to do this.
- According to the *Dietary Guidelines for Americans* (U.S. Department of Health and Human Services et al. 2005), most adults need about two to three 3-ounce servings of cooked meat or meat substitute per day based on calorie needs. Note: this might not be sufficient protein for children, pregnant, or lactating women, or larger than average-size adults.
- Encourage the purchase and consumption of protein foods that are lean and lower in saturated fat and cholesterol.
- Encourage the use of low-fat preparation methods.
- Encourage the use of measuring equipment to ensure serving sizes are in line with the relatively small amounts of meat being encouraged for healthy eating.

Educational points about fat

- Teach the foods (food groups) that provide fat. Teach that fat comes in some foods, such as meats, cheeses, and other dairy foods, such as ice cream. Fat, such as butter, margarine, mayonnaise, and salad dressing, is also added to foods. Because fat is a concentrated source of calories, its calories add up quickly. Limiting fat is an excellent way to limit calories. Use Table 3-3 to do this.

- Provide the number of fat grams or servings (5 grams of fat equals one serving) that is appropriate for the person and define a serving of fat. Refer to Table 3-1 to determine the appropriate grams or servings of fat for various calorie ranges.
- Encourage people to limit saturated fat intake by:
  - choosing lower-fat cheeses,
  - drinking fat-free milk and using fat-free yogurt and other dairy foods,
  - choosing lean red meats,
  - eating small servings of red meats,
  - using more fish than red meat.
- Encourage people to limit their intake of *trans* fat by limiting partially hydrogenated fat from commercially prepared foods. Note that decreasing sources of saturated fat will aid in decreasing *trans* fat.

CHAPTER FOUR

Concepts to Teach— Counting Carb, Reading Food Labels, and Measuring Portions

The concepts and teaching strategies from chapter 3 should provide a person learning carbohydrate counting with a solid foundation on general meal planning and personal nutrition. Once this foundation has been laid, more advanced concepts can be explored. This chapter will explore the last four concepts listed in the Assessment Checklist on page 14.

CONCEPTS TO TEACH

Know how to determine the carbohydrate counts of foods

People need resources to determine the carbohydrate counts of the variety of foods they eat. When initially teaching Basic Carbohydrate Counting, a handout that provides the serving sizes (within food groups) of commonly consumed foods might be sufficient. For example, 1/2 cup of starch, one small piece of fruit, 1 cup of milk, etc. Lists such as these are available in various American Diabetes Association (ADA) meal planning materials for educators, such as *Basic Carbohydrate Counting, The First Step in Diabetes Meal Planning, Choose Your Foods: Exchange Lists for Diabetes,* and others.

Educate people to pay attention to the carbohydrate count on the Nutrition Facts panel. Most people who eat a wide variety of foods, including restaurant foods, will need and learn to use additional carbohydrate counting resources, as exchanges/choices often don't match restaurant servings and options. More on the type of information available from restaurants and how to access these carbohydrate counts is available in chapter 10. Also note that Appendix I provides a listing of books, software, and online resources for carbohydrate counts of foods.

Some people who prepare recipes and enjoy cooking and baking may want to know how to obtain the carbohydrate counts of a serving of their favorite recipe. People can do this by using carbohydrate counting resources noted in Appendix I. They can get a carbohydrate count for all the ingredients in the recipe and then divide that total by the number of servings in the recipe. Some nutrient analysis websites listed in the carbohydrate counting resources in Appendix I allow people to perform this function online. Also, let people know that most diabetes-specific magazines and cookbooks provide the carbohydrate counts for their recipes.

If people are willing and able, encourage them to put together a chart or database with their Personal Carbohydrate Counts. Chapter 13 provides a process to teach people to accomplish this.

Know how to use the Nutrition Facts panel

Today, because of federal food and nutrition labeling regulations, nearly all packaged, canned, and prepared foods have a Nutrition Facts panel (Figure 4-1) on the food label (the only foods that generally do not are fresh fruits, vegetables, other fresh produce, and some fresh meat, poultry, and seafood). The total carbohydrate count is required on nearly all foods that have a Nutrition Facts panel. The Food and Drug Administration (FDA) website at www.fda.gov is a great resource for information on food labeling regulations. At the time of this writing, the direct link for food and nutrition labeling information is http://www.cfsan. fda.gov/label.html.

The following are teaching points about the Nutrition Facts panel in regard to Basic Carbohydrate Counting:

- The Nutrition Facts provide information based on one serving of the food. People need to take note of the panel serving and consider the portion they eat to correctly figure their carbohydrate count. Serving sizes on food labels are uniform and defined by the FDA. For example, one serving of bread is 30 grams and one serving of juice is 8 ounces. Servings must be noted in grams as well as household servings. For example, one slice, ten crackers, 8 ounces, etc. This makes the amounts easier to understand.
- Food label serving sizes are not necessarily the same as diabetes (or exchange/choice) servings. Table 3-4 (page 27) provides examples of how the servings can be the same or different.
- The total carbohydrate count includes all the components under total carbohydrate, including dietary fiber, sugars, and polyols (sugar alcohols). There is no need for people to pay special attention to sugars, as

they are counted as part of total carbohydrate. "Sugars" are defined by the FDA as both naturally occurring sugars and added sugars or all mono- and disaccharides (U.S. Food and Drug Administration 2004). Educators should explain that the word "sugars" on the food label is not just added sugars. This is often a point of confusion for people learning carbohydrate counting.

- Make sure that if people are doing meal planning according to servings that they know how to translate the grams of carbohydrate from a Nutrition Facts panel into a serving of food in their eating plan.

- The nutrition claims: sugar free, reduced sugars, and no added sugar or no sugar added do not mean the food is carbohydrate or calorie free. People still need to look at the amount of total carbohydrate and count it. (Chapter 10 provides additional information on polyols and how to teach people to fit these into their eating plan.)

Figure 4-1. Sample Nutrition Facts Panel

Nutrition Facts

Serving Size 1 cup (228g)
Servings Per Container 2

Amount Per Serving

Calories 260   **Calories from Fat** 120

	% Daily Value*
Total Fat 13g	**20%**
Saturated Fat 5g	**25%**
Trans Fat 2g	
Cholesterol 30mg	**10%**
Sodium 660mg	**28%**
Total Carbohydrate 31g	**10%**
Dietary Fiber 0g	**0%**
Sugars 5g	
Protein 5g	

Vitamin A 4%	•	Vitamin C 2%
Calcium 15%	•	Iron 4%

*Percent Daily Values are based on a 2,000 calorie diet. Your Daily Values may be higher or lower depending on your calorie needs.

	Calories:	2,000	2,500
Total Fat	Less than	65g	80g
Sat Fat	Less than	20g	25g
Cholesterol	Less than	300mg	300mg
Sodium	Less than	2,400mg	2,400mg
Total Carbohydrate		300g	375g
Dietary Fiber		25g	30g

Calories per gram:
Fat 9 • Carbohydrate 4 • Protein 4

Have and know how to use measuring equipment and other portion control tools

Teaching people what measuring equipment and portion control tools to have and how to use them is a critical aspect of teaching carbohydrate counting. Consider using the online tool from National Institutes of Health, called the Portion Distortion Quiz (*http://hp2010.nhlbihin.net/portion/* as of the time of this writing) to raise consciousness about the portions a person is currently eating.

The following is the measuring equipment that people should have at home and be encouraged to use regularly:

- Measuring cups for both liquids and solids
- Measuring spoons (a set)
- Food scale

Most will have the first two items, but not the scale. Encourage people to purchase an inexpensive scale ($10 to $15), particularly to measure foods that don't come with a Nutrition Facts panel, such as fresh fruit, fresh vegetables, bagels, and raw or cooked meats. More expensive food scales ($40 to $100) are also available. These scales may provide features such as the gram weight of the food and the grams of carbohydrate pulled from a database for several hundreds to thousands of common foods. The Diabetes Mall at www.diabetesnet. com or 800-988-4772 is a good resource for information on several of these scales. Additionally, the EatSmart Nutrition Scale (www.eatsmartscales.com) is a good choice.

Portion control tools are not just limited to measuring utensils. The following are additional portion control tools:

- *Nutrition Facts panel on food labels.* Encourage people to read the serving sizes on a food's Nutrition Facts panel. Make sure they realize that the nutrition information provided is for one reasonable serving of the food for most Americans. Have them think about the quantity they eat in comparison

Table 4-1. Hand Guides for Portion Control

Thumb tip = *1 teaspoon*
(from tip of finger to first knuckle)
Ex: 1 teaspoon mayonnaise or salad dressing

Thumb = *1 tablespoon*
(from tip of finger to second knuckle)
Ex: 1 ounce cheese or meat

Palm = *3 ounces*
Ex: 3 ounces cooked meat (boneless)

Tight fist or one open hand = *1/2 cup or 4 ounces of liquid*
Ex: one serving noodles, rice, or canned fruit or fruit juice

Open hand or two hands = *1 cup*
cupped together
Ex: 1 cup vegetables, 1 cup pasta

Note: Concern has been raised about the variation in hand sizes among people. Larger men will likely have larger hands than small women. This may be true, but hands are always at a person's side and it is likely that the person with larger hands has higher caloric needs.

Conversion from Raw to Cooked Meat

The weight difference between raw and cooked meat can sometimes be a point of confusion. To help people when they are selecting meat, provide the following guideline. Remind people that in restaurants, portions of meats, when noted, are provided in raw amounts. For example, a quarter pound hamburger equals about 3 ounces cooked and a 10-ounce T-bone steak equals about 6 ounces cooked.

- Raw meat without bone: use 4 ounces raw to get 3 ounces cooked.
- Raw meat with bone: use 5 ounces raw to get 3 ounces cooked.
- Raw poultry with skin and bone: use 4 1/4–4 1/2 ounces to get 3 ounces cooked. The extra 1/4–1/2 ounce accounts for the skin. (Remove the skin before or after cooking but before being eaten.)

to the food label portion. If willing, have them measure out this portion with measuring equipment, then put it into a serving item to see how the quantity looks.

- *Eyes.* Help people train their eyes to judge portions. Teach them that their eyes are always with them in the supermarket, at the bakery, or at restaurants. Tell people that the more they use measuring equipment at home, the better they will be at estimating portions when they eat out.
- *Hands.* Many educators find it helpful to teach the hand guides found in Table 4-1 to help people eat foods in proper portions. These can be particularly helpful for meals eaten away from home.

Additional portion control tips

While it is important to encourage people to use measuring equipment at home when possible, especially as they start to count carbohydrate, it is unrealistic to expect people to continue using these tools long term. For this reason it is important to provide additional portion control tips for eating at home and away from home.

Portion control tips for purchasing food and eating food at home:

- Keep measuring equipment—spoons, cups, and a scale—in an easy-to-use location. Consider weighing and measuring foods once a week. A reasonable suggestion may be to do it over the weekend, when a person may have more time.
- Use smaller plates and bowls. Less food looks like more food on smaller plates. People are less likely to overfill smaller plates.
- Encourage people not to serve family style. Putting bowls or platters of food on the table makes it easier to overeat.

- Put the leftovers (or what should be leftovers) away before eating.
- When buying produce—fruits, vegetables, and starches—buy the small pieces or plan to cut larger ones in half.
- When buying meat, fish, or poultry, purchase the amount needed for the meal, rather than too much. Give people examples. For instance, if a person is making hamburgers for four and wants 3-ounce cooked hamburgers, then only buy 16 ounces (1 pound) of meat. Or, if a person is buying turkey at the deli to make four sandwiches with 2 ounces of meat each, then buy as close to 1/2 pound as possible and make each sandwich with an equal amount of turkey.

Portion control tips for eating foods at a restaurant:

- Educate people about the words on menus or menu boards that mean large portions: giant, grande, supreme, extra large, jumbo, double, triple, double-decker, king size, and super.
- Educate people to seek out portion descriptors that mean small portions: junior, single, queen, petite, kiddie, and regular.
- Encourage people not to "super-size" or purchase meal deals, as these can promote overeating unless people are sharing parts of the meal, such as French fries. Teach that value equals being able to eat a healthy, reasonably portioned meal.
- Avoid all-you-can-eat restaurants or buffets as they encourage overeating.
- Teach "menu creativity" with restaurant menus. People don't automatically need to order a main course. They can order a soup and salad, an appetizer and soup, or a half portion. Encourage people to eat "family style" in a variety of restaurants—from American to ethnic (where it's more common). This type of "family style" eating encourages people to eat less by ordering fewer dishes than the number of people at the table and share the fewer menu items between diners. (This style of eating is in contrast to the portion control suggestion for eating at home that encourages people not to put large bowls of food on the table for sharing, or what's typically thought of as "family-style" service.)
- Encourage people and let them know it is okay to split, share, and mix and match menu items to get the foods they want in the portions they need.
- Show people how they can use the estimating capabilities they have gained as they have used their measuring and portion control equipment at home. Encourage the use of hand guides and well-trained eyes.
- Encourage assertiveness to ask for take-home containers, ideally at the start of the meal so the "second serving" can be put away before eating.

For further portion control education, use some of the following ideas and resources:

- Have samples of the type of measuring equipment people should have and use at home.
- Have plenty of Nutrition Facts panels from commonly eaten foods. Use these to help people determine proper portions.
- Have commonly sized bowls, plates, and cups that people have in their kitchens to show them how smaller quantities of foods look on dishes with which they are familiar.
- Use the above serving items to have people demonstrate their ability to measure foods accurately. Ask them to measure a nonperishable food, such as nuts or dry cereal, in a serving item and pour it into a measuring cup. Use a food model as an example for weighing meat or cheese.
- Use food models of fruit to demonstrate proper portions; people regularly don't count the amount of carbohydrate in fruit correctly.
- Consider purchasing and/or gathering additional portion control resources from the following sources (all websites as of the writing of this book):
  - The Idaho Plate Method (www.platemethod.com)
  - The Portion Doctor (www.portiondoctor.com)
  - NASCO (www.enasco.com/nutrition)
  - Nutrition Counseling and Education Services (www.ncescatalog.com)

Continually stress portion control

Educators need to continually reinforce the importance of eating proper portions and using measuring equipment and portion control tools. It is well known that people underestimate the amount of food they eat, whether they record this information or not. It is also easy to see how a person who is making many behavior changes and is eating healthier overall believes that eating larger portions of healthy foods will not make much difference. The reality is that slightly larger portions consumed every day do matter, especially for people who have minimal caloric needs. At the end of any day, extra grams of carbohydrate and calories can be the difference between achieving diabetes and nutrition goals or not.

Know how to interpret postprandial blood glucose levels

Checking and reviewing postprandial blood glucose levels regularly can provide healthcare providers and people with diabetes valuable insights into their glucose control. Postprandial levels often go unchecked and unanalyzed, usually because healthcare providers do not request them or because individuals already check so many fasting and mealtime levels that they don't want to check more.

Educators need to emphasize the value of postprandial monitoring, especially if A1C values are higher than expected, which could indicate people are likely missing high blood glucose levels after meals. Table I-1 on page 2 provides the goal for postprandial blood glucose and a note that postprandial levels should be checked 1–2 hours after the beginning of the meal.

If people who aren't on MDI or CSII therapy aren't willing to add more glucose checks, educators can encourage them to substitute a fasting or preprandial check for a postprandial check. People on MDI or CSII therapy, however, will need to add postprandial checks to their fasting and mealtime checks because they need this information for insulin dosing.

Encourage people to check postprandial blood glucose levels to accomplish the following:

- Gain more insights into blood glucose control after eating and before the next food intake
- Learn the impact of both the types of foods eaten and the amounts and make changes as needed
- Gain insights about the effectiveness of mealtime insulin dosing or other blood glucose–lowering medication and use the information to make changes in ICRs as needed
- Determine the duration of rapid-acting insulin action in order to individualize the bolus-on-board setting on insulin pumps or improve correction dosing using MDI

CHAPTER FIVE

Basic Carbohydrate Counting Case Studies

CASE STUDY #1: BENITA

Situation: Benita is a 47-year-old woman who owns her own health care consulting business. She is married and has one 10-year-old child. She was diagnosed with type 2 diabetes recently and was referred to a local diabetes education program. Benita had gestational diabetes in her only pregnancy and has struggled with her weight most of her adult life. She has gained 50 pounds over the years since her pregnancy. She has been on a host of diets over the years with little success. However, during her pregnancy, she did follow a meal plan to manage her gestational diabetes successfully.

Physical and Lab Data: Ht: 5′0″; Wt: 175 lb; BMI: 34; A1C: 7.4%; Hypertension is not under control; Total Cholesterol (TC): 225 mg/dl, HDL-C: 27 mg/dl, LDL-C: 132 mg/dl; Triglycerides (TG): 153 mg/dl

Blood Glucose–Lowering Medication(s): None

Food Habits/Daily Schedule:
Workdays:
- Wakes: 6 AM
- Breakfast: 7:30 AM: One whole banana and one bagel with cream cheese (eaten in her car on the way to work) or she skips breakfast. She drinks several cups of coffee with half and half and sugar throughout the morning.
- Lunch: 12:00 PM: Usually a restaurant meal—grilled chicken sandwich with French fries; tuna fish or chicken salad sandwich with potato chips; or

chef's salad. Once or twice a week, larger lunches out with clients.
- Evening meal: 7:30 PM: Home or in restaurants with clients or family. Her husband does the cooking. Meals at home generally contain salad, vegetable, starch, and meat. Benita notes that she probably eats too much because she is very hungry at this point. Meals in restaurants are often Italian, Continental, or Mexican food. She has trouble limiting portions in these settings.
- Evening snacking: Nibbles on chips or candy through the evening.

Weekends:
- Wakes: Later on the weekends.
- Breakfast: Time varies: Usually has a large breakfast.
- Lunch: Time varies: Often eats a light lunch of a meat sandwich.
- Evening meal: Time varies: Evening meal is often out at ethnic restaurants.

Physical Activity: She has just started walking her dogs again. Prior to this, however, she had done limited exercise.

Self-Monitoring Blood Glucose (SMBG): None to date.

Meal Planning: Benita worked with a dietitian during her pregnancy complicated by gestational diabetes. She was able to follow a meal plan during this time, but after the pregnancy went back to her old ways of eating. She wants to know how much carbohydrate she should eat at her meals and snacks. She realizes she needs to lose weight to control her blood glucose and other parameters.

Action Plan:

1. Benita was taught the basic concepts of carbohydrate counting by the dietitian in a one-on-one session. The dietitian provided Benita with carbohydrate intake goals (grams) for meals and one snack in the evening.

2. The dietitian reviewed Benita's current eating habits with her and provided suggestions for change to help her lose weight and eat healthier. She suggested Benita focus on portion control at home and in restaurants and provided a variety of tips.

3. The dietitian also encouraged Benita to use measuring equipment, particularly initially, to help her re-familiarize herself with proper portions.

4. Benita will attend the diabetes education center's class, Managing Type 2 Diabetes, to help her learn more about the elements of diabetes care and how to set goals to make behavior and lifestyle changes.

5. Benita was taught how to use a blood glucose meter and was encouraged to check her blood glucose two times a day at varied times before and one to two hours after she begins to eat her meals. The dietitian provided Benita with her target blood glucose goals.

Benita's Goals:

1. Eat about 45 grams of carbohydrate at breakfast and lunch and 60 grams at the evening meal each day.

2. Find and use measuring equipment to use when eating at home in order to learn to eat proper portions at home and in restaurants.

3. Use tips to control portions when in restaurants. Eat more salads for lunch. Do not order French fries or chips most days of the week.

4. Check blood glucose two times a day and record. Bring records to visit in one month.

Return Appointment with the Dietitian (One Month Later): Benita is pleased to report that her blood glucose levels are in her target ranges. Generally, her blood glucose is 90 to 100 mg/dl fasting and before meals. After meals her blood glucose ranges from 125 to 160 mg/dl. She has lost 4 pounds. Benita notes that she is focusing on weighing and measuring her carbohydrate foods and is really shocked at the small amounts she needs to eat to follow her carbohydrate counting plan. She is now drinking coffee with low-fat milk and a no-calorie sweetener and is choosing healthier options and smaller portions when she eats out. She notes that on the weekends she is less rigid with her food choices. This helps her not feel so restricted. Getting her walks in has been challenging. She is averaging a 15-minute walk about three days a week.

Educator Action Plan:

1. Applaud Benita for making many behavior changes, including learning SMBG, and learning more about how much she was previously eating. Encourage her to continue these positive behaviors.

2. Discuss strategies and develop a goal for increasing physical activity. Discuss the importance of physical activity in weight and diabetes control.

3. Reinforce the importance of continuing to weigh and measure foods. Encourage her to do this a couple times a week.

4. Discuss strategies for healthier snacking and eating on the weekends.

5. Let Benita know that her physician will be contacted and informed of her excellent progress. Inform her that her progress indicates that she does not currently need blood glucose–lowering medications, but this is likely to change over time, even with adherence to a healthy eating plan and sufficient physical activity. This is a common progression of type 2 diabetes.

CASE STUDY #2: MARY

Situation: Mary is a 52-year-old married woman who has been diagnosed with type 2 diabetes for four years. She works five days per week (Monday through Friday), from about 8:30 AM to 5:00 PM, as an office receptionist. Mary's family physician referred her to the diabetes education program at her local hospital. Mary wants to get her blood glucose levels in range and lose about 20 pounds.

Physical and Lab Data: Ht: 5′4″; Wt: 164 lb (weight has been stable within 3 pounds for eight years); BMI: 28; A1C: From 8.2% to 9.5% over the last two years; Hypertension controlled on medications; HDL-C: 34 mg/dl, LDL-C: 151 mg/dl; TG: 179 mg/dl

Blood Glucose–Lowering Medication(s):
- Before breakfast: 1000 milligrams metformin, 8 mg Amaryl (glimepiride)
- Before evening meal: 1000 milligrams metformin
- Mary's physician recently started her on 5 micrograms of exenatide (BYETTA) twice a day

Food Habits/Daily Schedule:
Workdays:
- Wakes: 7 AM; Meds: 7:30 AM
- Breakfast: 7:30 AM: 8 ounces orange juice, 1 1/2 cups cornflakes, 1 cup 2% milk, one whole banana, coffee with 2% milk and sugar substitute
- Lunch: 12:30 PM: 6-inch sub sandwich (ham and cheese or turkey and cheese) and 1 1/2-ounce bag potato chips or fast food hamburger and French fries (medium-size order), one large apple or orange (from home), diet soda
- Mid-afternoon snack: 3:00 PM: three small cookies, diet soda
- Evening meal: 6:30 PM: Tossed salad with 2 tablespoons regular dressing, 1 cup green or yellow vegetable, 2 cups rice, potatoes, or pasta, 6 ounces cooked beef, chicken, or fish.
- Bedtime snack: 9:30 PM: Either 1 cup light ice cream or frozen yogurt or 6 ounces yogurt with fruit

Workdays during week:
- Wakes: 8 AM; Meds: 8:30 AM
- Breakfast: 8:30 AM: Similar to workdays.
- Lunch: 12:30 PM: Frozen light entrée with piece of fruit.
- Mid-afternoon snack: 3:00 PM: Similar to workdays.
- Evening meal: 6:30 PM: Similar to workdays.
- Bedtime snack: 9:30 PM: Similar to workdays.

Weekends:
- Wakes: 8 AM; Meds: 8:30 AM
- Breakfast: 8:30 AM: Similar to workdays.
- Lunch: 12:30 PM: Frozen light entrée with piece of fruit.
- Mid-afternoon snack: 3:00 PM: Similar to workdays.
- Evening meal: 6:30 PM: Similar to workdays. Eats one or two evening meals out at Chinese, Italian, or Japanese restaurants. Might have glass of wine at meal and split a dessert.
- Bedtime snack: 9:30 PM: Similar to workdays.

Physical Activity: Moves around at work. Mary takes one 15 minute walk either before or after lunch. Weekends does gardening and housework.

SMBG: Checks one to two times per day—fasting and before evening meal. Average fasting: 160–220 mg/dl. Average pre-evening meal: 150–175 mg/dl.

Meal Planning: The only diabetes education Mary has had is one session with a dietitian at the hospital about one year after she was diagnosed. She was provided with a 1500-calorie meal plan and a booklet with diabetes exchanges. Mary notes she made a number of changes in her food choices and the portions she eats, but she is not able to follow the eating plan as she knows she should. She was frustrated by that meal plan because she didn't feel it provided information on the wide variety of foods she likes to eat. She is interested now in knowing how to fit a wider variety of foods into her eating plan, including convenience foods, restaurant foods, and sweets.

Action Plan:

1. Mary will attend the diabetes education center's class, Managing Type 2 Diabetes, to help her learn more about the elements of diabetes care and how to set goals to make behavior and lifestyle changes. This class also introduces Mary to the basic skills of carbohydrate counting, with the key message that eating a similar amount of carbohydrate at meals and snacks each day will help control blood glucose.

2. Mary will be provided with guidelines about how much carbohydrate to eat at her meals. She will be encouraged to limit her snacks to once a day. In class, Mary will write two sets of sample meals using the carbohydrate servings and grams she needs (see Table 3-2 on page 25).

3. Mary will learn how to use the Nutrition Facts panel information on foods to make decisions about buying and eating certain convenience and ready-to-eat foods.

4. Mary will be encouraged to weigh and measure her foods with measuring equipment. She will be provided with portion control tips for eating at home and in restaurants.

5. Mary will be encouraged to increase the frequency of her blood glucose monitoring to two to three times per day. She will be encouraged to check her fasting level and to begin to do some postprandial checking to detect the rise of blood glucose from meals.

Mary's Goals:

1. Get measuring equipment out and use it when eating at home to become more familiar with servings of foods.

2. Access and use web-based resources for carbohydrate counts of foods to learn the counts for foods she commonly eats, including restaurant foods.

3. Eat amounts of carbohydrate that are consistent with goal carbohydrate counts.

4. Check blood glucose two to three times a day and record. Bring records to visit in one month.

Final Diabetes Education Class (One Month Later): Mary is quite positive about the knowledge she has gained in class and the insights she now has about portion control and its effect on blood glucose. Mary has lost 3 pounds. Fasting blood glucose range is now 130–160 mg/dl, with postprandial levels range at 150–180 mg/dl.

Educator Action Plan:

1. Applaud Mary for making behavior changes and paying careful attention to portions. Encourage her to continue these positive behaviors.

2. With the Nutrition Facts panel labels from foods Mary regularly eats, have her figure the number of servings in a package.

3. With restaurant menus and nutrition information, discuss Mary's current choices, suggest healthier choices, and discuss strategies to decrease restaurant portions.

4. Discuss a goal to encourage more physical activity. Consider walking more and provide several strategies to increase energy expenditure in daily life.

5. Let Mary know that her physician will be contacted to encourage an increase in exenatide to 10 micrograms twice a day. She is tolerating well after one month on 5 micrograms of exenatide, her blood glucose levels have decreased nicely, but she is still not achieving target blood glucose goals.

CASE STUDY #3: DAVE

Situation: Dave is a 59-year-old widower who has had type 2 diabetes for 16 years. He is a retired mechanical engineer who volunteers at local schools and other community programs. He has a "lady friend" whom he sees several times a week. She prepares an evening meal for Dave a few nights a week or they go out to eat. Dave is currently frustrated with the swings of his blood glucose levels. He requested that his nurse practitioner refer him to a dietitian diabetes educator in the community who, according to his diabetes support group friends, teaches carbohydrate counting. Dave is willing to go and set up an appointment.

Physical and Lab Data: Ht: 5'10"; Wt: 198 lb (weight has increased slowly since retirement); BMI: 28; A1C: Last was 8.7%, up from usual 7.3 to 7.6%; Blood pressure under good control with medications; Blood lipids under good control with medications.

Blood Glucose–Lowering Medication(s):
- Before breakfast: 25 units insulin—75/25 (mix of 75% insulin lispro protamine suspension and 25% insulin lispro [rDNA origin]); Actos (pioglitazone hydrochloride)—45 mg
- Before evening meal: 20 units insulin—75/25 (mix of 75% insulin lispro protamine suspension and 25% insulin lispro [rDNA origin])

Food Habits/Daily Schedule:
Weekdays:
- Wakes: 8 AM; Meds: 8:15 AM
- Breakfast: 8:30 AM: Most mornings has 8 ounces orange juice, two packages

instant oatmeal, 1 tablespoon raisins, 1/2 cup 1% milk; or 8 ounce orange juice, 2 cup mixture of Cheerios, Mini Shredded Wheat, and All Bran with fiber, 1 cup 1% milk, one slice whole-wheat bread with butter. One morning a week has fast food sausage and egg on biscuit, or 2 donuts.

- Lunch: 12:30–1:30 PM: Most days packs two sandwiches with ham or turkey and cheese, small bag of chips, and large apple or banana. Sometimes has fast food hamburger or fried chicken sandwich with medium order of French fries and sugar-free iced tea or diet soda.
- Evening meal: 6:30–7:30 PM: Evening meals can be frozen entrée with meat, starch, and vegetable with dinner roll and salad; balanced meal made by "lady friend"—meat, starch, vegetable, salad with two glasses of wine (8–10 ounces total); or evening meal out at Italian, Mexican, Chinese, or American restaurant with a split dessert once or twice a week.
- Bedtime snack: 10:00–11:00 PM: Six sugar-free sandwich cookies or 1 cup sugar-free light ice cream.

Weekends:
- Schedule is similar to weekdays.

Physical Activity: Moves around when he volunteers at the school. In good weather, Dave takes about a 20-minute walk in his neighborhood two to three days a week. He does some gardening once or twice a week in good weather.

SMBG: Advised recently to check more often than first thing in the morning. He has been checking about three times a day both before and after some meals. His average fasting is 160–210 mg/dl, before lunch 60–140 mg/dl (some feelings of hypoglycemia when below 80 mg/dl), and after the evening meal 200–240 mg/dl.

Meal Planning: When Dave was diagnosed with diabetes, he and his wife were given an 1800-calorie meal plan by his doctor. They attended a series of classes for type 2 diabetes. Dave's wife kept up with his meal plan before she became ill, but Dave never understood it that well. He thought of it as his wife's job. Dave believed that as long as he ate his meals on time he would be fine. When Dave's wife became ill, eating healthy or eating on time became more difficult. After Dave's wife died, this became even more difficult. He began eating more convenience foods, restaurant foods, and fast food meals. These eating habits led to weight gain and diminishing blood glucose control.

Dietitian's Action Plan:

1. The dietitian believes Dave and his "lady friend" have the ability to learn Basic Carbohydrate Counting.

2. Dave's knowledge of carbohydrates and servings is minimal at present. To build Dave's knowledge, the dietitian teaches Dave the skills of Basic Carbohydrate Counting. She provides information with the carbohydrate counts of common foods and encourages him to purchase a book with carbohydrate counts for more foods or to access one of the websites listed in the carbohydrate counting resources she provided (see Appendix I).

3. The dietitian provides Dave with the amount of carbohydrate to eat at meals and a snack before bed.

4. The dietitian suggests that Dave begin to weigh and measure foods when he eats at home to get a feel for how much he really eats. She teaches him the hand guide (see page 34) to estimate portions away from home and in restaurants. They also review healthier choices in fast food restaurants.

5. The dietitian provides Dave with a form to record his carbohydrate and blood glucose results (Appendix III). He is to keep food, carbohydrate counts, and blood glucose records for two weeks and fax them in. They have scheduled a phone conversation for two weeks and a follow-up appointment for one month.

Dave's Goals:

1. Using his carbohydrate goals, develop two sample meals for breakfast, lunch, and the evening meal.

2. Using food labels and web-based resources provided by the dietitian, gather the carbohydrate counts for several of the convenience and restaurant foods he eats.

3. Weigh and measure foods when he eats the evening meal at home. Dave will ask his "lady friend" to do this at her house as well.

4. Check blood glucose levels three to four times a day, rotating between before and after meals.

5. Record carbohydrate intake and blood glucose results on provided form. Fax in records in time for phone conversation in two weeks.

Follow-Up by Telephone Two Weeks Later:

1. Dave and the dietitian both notice that his blood glucose levels are down about 10 to 20 mg/dl overall. Dave has had an increase in the frequency of mild hypoglycemia before lunch and before bed.

2. The dietitian notes she will contact Dave's nurse practitioner and suggest that Dave might do better on a bedtime injection of Lantus (insulin glargine; see action curves on page 150) and varied doses of rapid-acting insulin before meals, based on the amount of carbohydrate he eats. She believes this will diminish the hypoglycemia he is having as his blood glucose control improves. This regimen, while more complex, will provide Dave with more flexibility in terms of food choices and in the timing of his meals.

3. After weighing and measuring his food more often and researching carbohydrate counts, Dave observes that he has been overeating.

Individual counseling one month later:

1. The dietitian let Dave know that the nurse practitioner agreed to have her work with Dave to change his insulin regimen and, when he is ready, he should set up a visit with the nurse practitioner to do so. The nurse practitioner also agreed to have the dietitian teach Dave, if she assessed he was able, to use rapid-acting insulin prior to each of his meals based on his preprandial blood glucose level and his insulin-to-carbohydrate ratio (ICR). They discussed how Advanced Carbohydrate Counting would be more work, but could help Dave achieve better glucose control and also gain greater flexibility in his food choices and the timing of his meals. Also, he will not have to eat a nighttime snack.

2. The dietitian assessed that Dave was keeping good records and was checking his blood glucose about three times a day. She asked if he would be willing to check his preprandial blood glucose more frequently, and possibly start checking two hours after beginning a meal to determine the effect of the rapid-acting insulin.

3. From Dave's food records, the dietitian noted that Dave was doing a good job approximating the amount of carbohydrate he was eating, but he was still eating more carbohydrate than he needed. Also, he had not been successful making his fast food or other restaurant choices and continued to overeat.

Advanced Carbohydrate Counting

CHAPTER SIX

Concepts to Teach— Advanced Carbohydrate Counting

Once a person has developed an understanding of Basic Carbohydrate Counting, it should be determined whether or not it is advantageous to progress education to the more advanced concepts and strategies of Advanced Carbohydrate Counting. The person progressing to Advanced Carbohydrate Counting should be using or transitioning to a diabetes medication regimen that will make the knowledge and use of Advanced Carbohydrate Counting advantageous for their lifestyle and diabetes control. Generally this includes multiple daily injection (MDI) or continuous subcutaneous insulin infusion pump (CSII). For example, Advanced Carbohydrate Counting is appropriate for a person like the case study Dave (see chapter 5), who has type 2 diabetes and is transitioning his insulin therapy from twice-a-day injections of 75/25 insulin to an MDI regimen with long-acting and rapid-acting insulin. Advanced Carbohydrate Counting would also be useful for a person such as Barbara (a case study discussed later in chapter 9), who is transitioning from an MDI regimen with long-acting and rapid-acting insulin to CSII.

People who are ready to progress to learn and use Advanced Carbohydrate Counting should be able to demonstrate that they have the knowledge and skills of Basic Carbohydrate Counting listed in the Assessment Checklist from chapter 2 (see page 14) and discussed in chapters 3 and 4. In addition, the educator needs to feel confident that the person and/or the family member(s) or caretakers responsible for the person's diabetes care will be able to accumulate the knowledge and perform the necessary skills for Advanced Carbohydrate Counting detailed in this chapter.

ADVANCED CARBOHYDRATE COUNTING CONCEPTS

Advanced Carbohydrate Counting knowledge and skills are generally more demanding and include understanding of the following concepts:

☐ Insulin action—onset, peak, and duration
☐ Insulin regulation for 24-hour blood glucose control
☐ Basal (background) insulin and bolus (food coverage) insulin
☐ Correction bolus insulin
☐ Insulin delivery vehicles (syringes, pens, pumps)
☐ Calculation of insulin-to-carbohydrate ratio (ICR)
☐ Calculation of correction factor (CF) and correction or supplemental doses
☐ Determination of meal and snack (preprandial) bolus insulin doses
☐ Use of pattern management to determine medication adjustments
☐ Use of customized ICR(s) to adjust meal and snack medication doses
☐ Use of customized CF(s) to correct hyperglycemia or use of CF(s) in reverse to prevent hypoglycemia
☐ Understanding the importance of checking blood glucose levels at least four times per day (before meals) and, on occasion, postprandially and during the night
☐ Correcting hyperglycemia
☐ Correcting hypoglycemia (including prevention and treatment)
☐ The need to consistently carry necessary medications, supplies (including delivery device) to use medications, and hypoglycemia treatment aids

Insulin action

People who use MDI or CSII therapy need to be well versed in the action curves—onset, action, peak, and duration—of the insulins they take (see chapter 12). Educators should not assume that people know the action curves of the insulins they take. A simple drawing of action curves can help people understand the interrelationship between their insulin regimen and carbohydrate intake. Other teaching aids and resources for health professionals to show insulin action profiles are available from insulin manufacturers and other sources.

Insulin regulation for 24-hour blood glucose control

With the advent of rapid- and long-acting insulin analogs, it is possible for people with diabetes to attempt to mimic the natural pattern of basal and bolus insulin with exogenous insulin(s). Exogenous replacement of amylin, a hormone cosecreted with insulin that suppresses inappropriate postprandial gluagon secretion and slows gastric emptying, with its analog, pramlintide, is also available and can be used by adults with type 1 diabetes as well as adults with type 2 diabetes who use mealtime insulin.

For most people with type 1 diabetes, the concept of MDI and "basal-bolus" insulin has become the preferred insulin therapy regimen. This is also true for many people with type 2 diabetes who use insulin, though not as universal. This therapy consists of one or two injections of intermediate- or long-acting basal insulin along with rapid- or short-acting bolus insulin. Premixed insulin combinations, such as 70/30, 75/25, or 50/50 (a mix of 75%, 70%, or 50% NPH or insulin lispro protamine and 30%, 25%, or 50% insulin lispro, insulin aspart, or regular) are not appropriate or useful for people who adjust bolus insulin for carbohydrate counting. (See Figures 12-4, 12-5, 12-6, and 12-7 in chapter 12, pages 150–152.)

Basal (background) insulin

Basal (background) insulin reduces hepatic glucose production, and, if appropriately dosed, helps to achieve and maintain fasting, between-meal, and nocturnal target glycemic levels. In MDI therapy, basal insulin can be twice-daily injections of intermediate-acting insulin, or once- or twice-daily injections of long-acting insulin. In CSII, basal insulin is usually rapid-acting (but sometimes regular) insulin that is continuously infused 24 hours per day in small incremental doses and individualized based on need. Basal insulin usually accounts for about 50% of a person's total daily dose (TDD), but can range from 40–60% of their TDD (Bolderman 2002; Walsh and Roberts 2006).

Bolus (food coverage and correction dose) insulin

Insulin that is injected or infused to "cover" the carbohydrate eaten at meals or snacks is bolus insulin. In intensive diabetes management, bolus insulin is regular or rapid-acting insulin and a specific, individualized dose of insulin is delivered at the meal or snack to match the amount of carbohydrate consumed. The bolus dose is based primarily on the person's individual ICR(s). People may have more than one ICR depending on several factors, such as time of day, illness, menses, etc.

The convenience of injecting or infusing insulin at the start of, during, or after the meal to cover the precise amount of carbohydrate eaten allows for more precise dosing with resultant postprandial target glycemia. For this reason, rapid-acting insulin is usually the bolus insulin of choice, although there are circumstances, such as with infants and toddlers or with the presence of gastroparesis, that may warrant the use of regular insulin as the preferred prandial insulin. In addition to prandial insulin, bolus insulin may also be in the form of correction doses to decrease hyperglycemia. Bolus insulin usually accounts for about 50% of a person's TDD, but can range from 40% to 60%.

Factors to consider in the calculation of a bolus dose include:

- Amount of carbohydrate
- Current blood glucose level
- Target blood glucose level
- ICR
- CF (if correction bolus dose)
- Amount of insulin remaining from most recent bolus ("insulin on board")
- Exercise
- Alcohol
- Stress
- Illness

For specifics on reviewing blood glucose records and insulin bolus coverage, refer to chapter 8.

Insulin delivery vehicles

It's important to discuss insulin delivery options and provide guidelines for insulin delivery that make it appropriate, comfortable, and convenient for the person. As of the time of this printing, there are four available vehicles for insulin delivery: syringes, pens, pumps, and jet injectors.

Syringes

Plastic disposable insulin syringes vary in their volume capacity, needle gauge, and needle length. Syringes are available in 1/3-, 1/2-, and 1-cc capacity. For doses <30 units, a 1/3-cc syringe is best. Needle lengths vary from 5/16-inch to 1/2-inch and are available in 27-, 28-, 29-, 30-, and 31-gauge widths. The higher the gauge number, the thinner the needle and the greater the comfort.

Insulin pens

Insulin pens, introduced in the United States in 1987, provide added convenience and are available with different needle lengths and gauges. Insulin pens are the size of a thick marking pen and can be disposable (containing factory-installed prefilled pen cartridges) or refillable using prefilled insulin pen cartridges. The cartridges hold either 150 or 300 units. Both disposable and refillable insulin pens use disposable pen needles, ranging in length from 3/16-inch to

1/2-inch. Pen needle gauge sizes range from 29 to 31. An advantage of insulin pen therapy is click- or dial-unit dosing that assures greater accuracy and convenience. However, since pens contain insulin-filled cartridges, storage may be a concern. Insulin pen manufacturers recommend storing opened pens at room temperature based on the type of insulin, and storage times vary from 10, 14, or 28 days. Unopened insulin pens, like insulin vials, should be stored in the refrigerator and are good up to their expiration date.

Both insulin syringes and insulin pens are available with half-unit markings. Half-unit markings may be helpful for those who use small doses; generally, the accuracy of half-unit doses is better with pens than with syringes (Keith, Nicholson, and Rogers 2004).

Insulin pump

An insulin pump most closely mimics physiological insulin replacement and provides the greatest amount of flexibility and accuracy for insulin dosing. Chapter 7 provides more detail on insulin pumps and CSII.

Jet injectors

Jet, or air, injectors are also available for insulin delivery and may appeal to people who fear needles, including both children and adults. Insulin delivery with the use of a jet injector can be as precise as delivery via a syringe or pen, but jet injectors are more costly than syringes and pens (but less costly than an insulin pump) and may not be covered by insurance. Proper training to determine individualized pressure settings can prevent jet injector skin bruising. Jet injector use is not as common as traditional insulin syringes, pens, and pumps.

Calculation of ICR(s)

The ICR is a personalized ratio of how much carbohydrate is covered by units of insulin, usually expressed as $u:c$, where u represents units of insulin (almost always 1) and c represents grams of carbohydrate. A person's ICR depends on their sensitivity to insulin. Generally, the more sensitive someone is to insulin, the larger the amount of carbohydrate covered by one unit of insulin. Also, because some people are more or less insulin-resistant at different times of the day or month or have different levels of activity during the day, they might need more than one ICR. People who experience a dawn phenomenon, for example, may require a breakfast ICR that is higher than a ratio used during the remainder of the day (i.e., more insulin is needed at breakfast to cover the same amount of carbohydrate consumed at other times of the day).

The ICR can be calculated using any of the various methods detailed below. Use whichever method seems most appropriate based on the information at hand. If possible, use one method to calculate a person's ICR, and then use another method to compare or validate the ratio.

It is important to note that if the person's basal insulin dose(s) is incorrect, the process of determining the person's ICR will take longer and will yield inconsistent results. For people who use an insulin pump, it is best to evaluate and determine the person's correct basal rates before trying to fine-tune, tweak, or determine the appropriate ICR(s). *The basal insulin dose(s) or rates must be correct, or the ICR(s) and CF(s) will not work* (Bolderman 2002).

Hidden Carbs

Accurate assessment of consumed carbohydrates is essential to MDI therapy. A common complication is incorrect accounting of "hidden" or overlooked carbohydrate. Remind people that even the smallest amount of carbohydrate (such as 5 grams) can affect their glucose levels, especially if they are more insulin resistant and have an ICR in the range of 1:10 or less. Inappropriate calculation of hidden carbohydrate, such as the breading on a chicken filet patty or corn starch and sugar in the sauce of a Chinese dish, can result in under bolusing to cover a meal. Accordingly, when carbohydrate is not covered with the appropriate matched dose of bolus insulin, glucose excursions will result. Remind people to be cognizant of the carbohydrate in:

- Bread/rolls from the bread basket in a restaurant eaten while waiting for the meal
- Breading on a chicken patty or fish filet
- Breading on meat/poultry/vegetable in fast food or ethnic meals
- Meal components, such as cornstarch in mixed dishes and soups
- Soup base in creamed or some ethnic soups (e.g., egg drop)
- Pasta sauce or tomato sauce in an Italian meal
- Barbecue sauce (e.g., on ribs)
- Croutons in salad
- Large amounts of salad dressing
- Larger-than-usual sandwich roll
- Larger-than-usual sub roll
- Icing on cake or cupcake
- Pie crust
- Doughnut fillings, such as jelly or cream
- Alcoholic beverage mixers, including juice, regular soda, and non-diet tonic water
- Beer and wine

Method #1: Food diary, insulin bolus dose, and self-monitoring blood glucose (SMBG) information

Ask the person to keep at least one week of self-monitoring blood glucose (SMBG) records, including:

- Fasting, preprandial, and 1- to 2-hour (after the start of the meal) postprandial glucose (PPG) results
- Preprandial bolus insulin doses
- Amount of carbohydrate consumed at meals, snacks, and other times, such as for hypoglycemia treatment (it is helpful for people to eat the same amount of carbohydrate for breakfasts, lunches, evening meals, and snacks during the week of keeping records)
- Exercise, illness, stress, menses, and alcohol consumption, including times and other related details of these factors (such as duration and intensity of exercise, pre/onset/duration of menses, amount of alcohol, etc.)

With these records, determine the amount of insulin the person used to cover the amount of carbohydrate consumed at each meal by dividing the total grams of carbohydrate by the number of units of insulin (Bolderman 2002). The result is the amount of carbohydrate covered by 1 unit of insulin, expressed as the ICR of one unit to x grams of carbohydrate.

Example:

- Preprandial blood glucose within target range
- Consumed 66 grams of carbohydrate
- Used 6 units of bolus insulin (rapid- or short-acting)
- 2-hour PPG is within target range
- $66 \div 6 = 11$
- ICR is 1 unit of insulin to 11 grams of carbohydrate, or 1:11

This method is most effective if the person's SMBG records indicate that he or she is consistently within preprandial and PPG target range. If blood glucose is generally not in control, or carbohydrate intake is varied, or there are too many other factors that affect blood glucose levels during the record-keeping time, this method may not produce an accurate ICR.

Method #2: The Rule of 500

This method, widely used by clinicians to determine ICRs, is based on TDD of insulin divided into 500. The result is the amount of carbohydrate that one unit of rapid-acting insulin will cover (returning levels to target range) in about

3–4 hours postprandially, or that one unit of short-acting insulin will cover in about 5–6 hours postprandially. Some clinicians find that dividing 450 (rather than 500) by the TDD is more accurate for insulin and/or for people who are less sensitive to insulin.

Example:

- Basal insulin dose: 8 units insulin glargine twice daily
- Bolus insulin doses: insulin aspart pre-breakfast 5 units; pre-lunch 6 units; pre-dinner 7 units
- TDD = 8 + 8 + 5 + 6+ 7 = 34 units
- Fasting, preprandial, and 2-hour PPG values are within target range
- 500 ÷ 34 = 14.7 (round to 15)
- ICR is 1 unit to 15 grams of carbohydrate, or 1:15

Currently, some clinicians are using other formulas and calculation methods based on their research. For example, the formula: (217/TDD) + 3 = ICR (King 2007).

Example:

- TDD is 34 units
- 217 ÷ 34 = 6.38
- 6.38 + 3 = 9.38, round to 10
- ICR is 1 unit to 10 grams of carbohydrate, or 1:10

Method #3: Using a formula based on weight and TDD

Using body weight and TDD is yet another way to determine an ICR. Using this method, multiply the person's body weight in pounds (BW) by 2.8 and then divide the result by the TDD, giving the formula (BW)2.8/TDD = ICR (Davidson et al. 2003).

Example:

- BW is 168 pounds and TDD is 38 units
- 168 × 2.8 = 470.4 ÷ 34 = 13.8 (round to 14)
- ICR is 1 unit to 14 grams of carbohydrate, or 1:14

Method #4: Using the CF to calculate the ICR

Once a person's CF is calculated (see section below, Calculation of CF and correction or supplemental insulin dose), multiplying it by 0.33 is another way to calculate an ICR.

Examples:

- CF is 60 mg/dl
- $60 \times 0.33 = 19.8$ (round to 20)
- ICR is 1 unit to 20 grams of carbohydrate, or 1:20

- CF is 50 mg/dl
- $50 \times 0.33 = 16.5$ (round to 17)
- ICR is 1 unit to 17 grams of carbohydrate, or 1:17

- CF is 45 mg/dl
- $45 \times 0.33 = 14.8$ (round to 15)
- ICR is 1 unit to 15 grams of carbohydrate, or 1:15

Other considerations

Deriving the ICR by the above methods is merely a starting point. Using different methods with the same parameters yields different results, so many clinicians calculate the ICR using the average of two or three methods. Some clinicians begin by assuming an ICR of 1:15 for most adults and a ratio of 1:20 or 1:25 for most children, as children tend to be more insulin-sensitive. However, because a person's insulin needs and sensitivities vary based on age and life situations (refer to Table 6-1 on page 63), it is best to spend a few extra minutes individually calculating these factors.

Detailed records of SMBG results, carbohydrate intake, and insulin doses provide useful information to make ratio adjustments. Some people need different ratios for different times of the day, and women may need different ratios at different phases of the menstrual cycle. Remind people to recalculate their ICR and use their new ratio if:

- TDD changes by more than a couple of units
- Body weight changes more than a few pounds
- Lifestyle changes create different amounts or types of physical activity, stress, or changes in sleeping hours (such as time zone changes)

Adjusting the ICR

To correct postprandial hypoglycemia or hyperglycemia (assuming the background or basal insulin dose(s) is correct), the ICR may need to be adjusted. Chapter 8 provides more detail on this subject.

Calculation of CF and correction or supplemental insulin dose

The insulin CF is defined as the amount of blood glucose (in mg/dl) lowered by 1 unit of rapid- or short-acting insulin. Although different names are used—correction factor (CF), insulin sensitivity factor, or supplemental factor—this is the method universally used for calculating the amount of insulin needed to return blood glucose to within the preprandial target range.

Two commonly accepted formulas are used as starting points in determining the CF: The 1500 Rule and The 1800 Rule. More recently, additional "rules" have come into practice: The 2000 Rule, The 1700 Rule, and a modified CF Rule. All of these Rules apply a mathematical constant that expresses the relationship between body size and insulin action.

The 1500 Rule was originally developed in the 1970s by endocrinologist Paul C. Davidson, MD, FACE, for calculating CF with short-acting insulin. Using regular insulin and Biostator data, people whose TDD was 50 units were found to have a reduction of 30 mg/dl with one unit of regular insulin. Thus, it was found that dividing the constant 1500 (or 50 × 30) by TDD would produce a reasonable CF estimate. With the introduction of rapid-acting insulin in the 1990s, John Walsh, PA, CDE, a pump specialist (Walsh and Roberts 2006), modified The 1500 Rule into The 1800 Rule.

Dr. Davidson and his colleagues have since developed a mathematical model based on data from nearly 500 pump patients in their practice. Dr Davidson modified his 1500 Rule to The 1700 Rule in 2003. The 1700 Rule is one part of the statistical estimates used by Dr. Davidson and his colleagues to determine insulin pump therapy formulas. These are known as The AIM (Accurate Insulin Management) Formulas (Davidson, Steed, and Bode 2003).

Examples:
The 1800 Rule

- TDD is 34 units
- 1800 ÷ 34 = 52.9 (round up to 53, but it may be easier to round up to 55 or 60—always round up when calculating a CF)
- CF is 53 (or 55 or 60) mg/dl: one unit of rapid-acting insulin decreases glucose 55 mg/dl

The 1700 Rule

- TDD is 34 units
- 1700 ÷ 34 = 50
- CF is 50 mg/dl: one unit of rapid-acting insulin decreases glucose 50 mg/dl

The 1500 Rule

- TDD is 34 units
- 1500 ÷ 34 = 44 (round up to 45 or 50)
- CF is 45 mg/dl: one unit of short-acting insulin decreases glucose 45 mg/dl

John Walsh, PA, CDE, modified his 1800 Rule to The 2000 Rule. Walsh found that The 2000 Rule works well and is a bit more cautious, yielding a slightly smaller number of units for correction boluses (Walsh and Roberts 2006).

In 2006, based on his research, Allen B. King, MD, FACP, FACE, CDE, proposed a different rule for calculating the correction factor: (1076/TDD) + 12 = CF. Dr. King maintains that his modification more closely determines a person's correction factor (Evert 2006).

King's modification rule

- TDD is 34 units
- 1076 ÷ 34 = 31.64 + 12 = 43.64 (round up to 45)
- CF is 45 mg/dl: one unit of rapid-acting insulin decreases glucose 45 mg/dl.

These "rules" suggest calculating the CF based on the following:

- The 1500 Rule—for people who use short-acting (regular) insulin or are insulin-resistant
- The 1700, 1800, or 2000 Rule—for people who use rapid-acting insulin analogs or are insulin-sensitive
- King's 2006 rule is (1076 ÷ TDD) + 12 = CF

Keep in mind that since these rules use the TDD of insulin, the resulting factor is a reflection of overall blood glucose control. *If control is not optimal, the TDD can be an indication of too much, too little, or inappropriate distribution of insulin between the basal and bolus amounts. No matter which rule is used, recalculate the CF if the TDD changes more than a few units. Consider the use of these rules as dosing starting points and then fine-tune ICR and CF based on blood glucose results and patterns.*

Correction or supplemental insulin dose

A correction, or supplemental insulin, dose uses a person's CF to determine the amount of rapid- or short-acting insulin taken to return an elevated blood glucose level to target level. It is important to identify *individualized* pre- and postprandial target blood glucose goals for and with each person. These targets will be used to determine the correction dose of insulin by providing a way to measure how much blood glucose is above or below target. Review the target blood glucose goals in Table I-1 on page 2. There are several methods used to calculate a correction dose.

One unit per 50 mg/dl

Using this method, one unit of rapid- or short-acting insulin is administered to lower blood glucose by 50 mg/dl. This is a commonly used starting point, but may not be appropriate for everyone. Clinicians may use a starting point of 100 mg/dl for children or insulin-sensitive adults.

Sliding scale

This method provides a guideline for the number of units of rapid- or short-acting insulin to use based on the blood glucose range that needs to be corrected. This was once popular, but has grown out of acceptance by many clinicians for its lack of precision and inability to be individualized (Hirsch and Hirsch 2001).

Example using the sliding scale:
Blood glucose 100–150 mg/dl: add 1 unit
Blood glucose 151–200 mg/dl: add 2 units

The 2000, 1800, 1700, or 1500 Rule

These or other recently developed rules (see section above) that are based on a person's CFs (people may need more than one) allow a greater amount of

CSII Correction Dosing

People who use an insulin pump (CSII) are able to add the precise amount of calculated insulin for a correction dose. Most of the current generation of insulin pumps, known as "smart pumps," can also take into account the remaining activity of insulin from the most recent bolus dose to correct high blood glucose or all insulin on board from the most recent food and correction bolus. This is known as insulin on board or bolus on board.

If there is active insulin still on board based on the duration of insulin action set by the user, the pump will suggest a reduced amount of correction insulin. It is important for clinicians to realize that each pump company applies a unique calculation to derive the insulin on board. The setting for duration of insulin action should be individualized by the clinician and pump user. Generally, clinicians use between 3 and 4 hours for duration of insulin action. Some pumps allow increments of 30 minutes and others only allow increments of 1 hour. Chapter 7 provides more detail on CSII.

individualization, but again, are based on a person's TDD of insulin, which may or may not be indicative of optimal control.

Example using the CF:

- Preprandial blood glucose is 277 mg/dl
- Target blood glucose level is 100 mg/dl
- CF is 60 mg/dl
- 277 − 100 = 177 mg/dl above target level
- 177 ÷ 60 = 2.95
- Correction dose of insulin is 3 units (2.95 units if using an insulin pump; see box CSII Correction Dosing)

Other considerations

For those following MDI regimens or those who use CSII without "smart pump" functionality, cognizance of "on board" insulin—insulin that may still be active from previous injections or infusions—is vital to prevent hypoglycemia. Reinforce the need to consider the timing of the most recent meal or correction dose when calculating a correction dose based on the current blood glucose level.

Other factors that should be considered are physical activity, stress, illness, and the amount and timing of alcohol consumption. All these factors can affect a person's sensitivity to insulin.

A correction factor can also range greatly from individual to individual. For an adult with type 1 diabetes, 1 unit of rapid-acting insulin may decrease blood glucose 60 mg/dl, while for an insulin-resistant person with type 2 diabetes, 1 unit of rapid-acting insulin may decrease the blood glucose only 20 mg/dl. It is important to individualize the CF and to recheck its accuracy periodically when there are TDD or lifestyle changes. See Table 6-1 for general guidelines on insulin sensitivity tendencies.

Table 6-1. Stages of Life and Life Situations: Insulin Sensitivity and Insulin Resistance

Insulin sensitive	*Insulin resistant*
Children with type 1 diabetes	Children in puberty
Lean people with type 1 diabetes	People with type 2 diabetes
Conditioned athletes	Late-term pregnant women
Newly diagnosed with type 1 diabetes	People ill with an infection
	People on steroids
	People experiencing high stress levels

Determination of meal and snack (preprandial) bolus insulin doses

In many ways, determining a proper preprandial insulin dose, one that accurately covers ingested carbohydrate and results in target postprandial blood glucose levels, is a primary aim of Advanced Carbohydrate Counting. Calculating this dose often draws on many of the skills and concepts discussed above, including accurate carbohydrate counting, SMBG, ICRs, and correction doses based on personalized CFs.

To determine the preprandial insulin dose, an accurate assessment of prandial carbohydrate must first be made. Next, individuals must use their ICR to determine the amount of insulin necessary to cover their meal or snack. Then, following a preprandial blood glucose check, they must determine if an additional correction dose is necessary to return glucose to target levels. If the preprandial blood glucose level is within the target range, no correction bolus is needed. If preprandial blood glucose is below target range, a smaller preprandial bolus may be needed. Review chapter 8.

Example:

- Target blood glucose level is 100 mg/dl
- ICR is 1:12
- CF is 40 mg/dl
- Preprandial blood glucose level is 237 mg/dl
- 60 grams of carbohydrate are to be consumed
- 60 ÷ 12 = 5 units of insulin to cover the carbohydrate
- 237 mg/dl – 100 mg/dl = 137 mg/dl above target level
- 137 mg/dl ÷ 40 = 3.4 units of insulin to decrease the preprandial elevated blood glucose
- 5 units + 3.4 units = 8.4 units of insulin (insulin pump bolus) or round down to 8 units of insulin if using syringe, pen, or jet injector

It is important that the blood glucose check used to determine insulin doses are preprandial and not postprandial. A one- or two-hour postprandial blood glucose measurement reflects the action of the previous preprandial dose of rapid- or short-acting insulin, which is not yet complete (see Duration of Insulin Action in chapter 7). If a postprandial glucose measure is used to calculate a correction dose, there is the possibility of administering too much insulin and causing hypoglycemia. Encourage people to space meals at least three to four hours apart, and to make sure that the dose they are calculating is based on a true preprandial blood glucose level.

It is important to reiterate the significance of on-board insulin. People are often confused by hypoglycemia that can occur when a pre-snack or correction bolus of rapid-acting insulin is administered three to five hours after their last correction bolus. This hypoglycemia can occur because people haven't factored in the remaining action of insulin, and therefore blood glucose–lowering effect, from the first dose. This is commonly referred to as "insulin stacking" (Hirsch 2005).

People need to be taught that rapid-acting insulin has, most commonly, in the range of three to four hours of action. They need to account for the remaining insulin on board if they take additional rapid-acting insulin within the duration of action from the previous dose. Teach people to get in the habit of asking themselves, "When did I take my last bolus dose(s) and was it within three to four hours of the bolus dose that I'm about to take?" If the answer is no, then the dose should be based on a higher or postprandial blood glucose target (such as 160 to 180 mg/dl). Some clinicians teach people to use the following rule of thumb to prevent insulin stacking: *Do not bolus for a high blood glucose reading within three to four hours of the last bolus.* If possible, the number of hours of action for rapid-acting insulin should be individually determined. One way to do this is to ask the person to take a preprandial bolus to cover a meal with an easy-to-determine amount of carbohydrate. Then the blood glucose should be checked every hour for five hours. The point when the blood glucose hits a nadir and starts to rise back up is a practical estimate of duration of action. This method makes the assumption that the person's basal insulin dose or rates are set accurately. Due to variables on any given day, it is best to conduct this test on several occasions to derive an average.

PRACTICAL ADVICE ON BOLUS DOSE TIMING FOR PEOPLE USING RAPID-ACTING INSULIN

Many experts agree, based on research and experience, that to help people achieve optimal pre- and postprandial blood glucose control, rapid-acting insulin should ideally be taken at least 10 to 15 minutes before food consumption when blood glucose is in a preprandial target range. Health care professionals know, however, that the ideal isn't always the reality, and people need practical advice for everyday living. The following practical tips may help people who practice intensive diabetes management and use either MDI or CSII. Make sure that people to whom you provide these practical tips have sufficient knowledge and competence to apply the information, and that they use these tips only when their ICR(s), CF(s), and other parameters have been established.

Many of these practical tips are easier and more convenient to implement if people use an insulin pen or insulin pump for bolus doses. Encourage people who are willing and able to use these insulin delivery devices to do so, and advocate on the patients' behalf for their use to the appropriate diabetes health care providers.

Stay ahead of blood glucose rise (be proactive rather than reactive)

There is agreement among health care professionals that it is easier to keep blood glucose in control by providing enough insulin to cover food than it is to be reactive and treat an elevated blood glucose level that occurs because of lack of sufficient insulin given at the correct time. This is an important point to make to people practicing intensive diabetes management. People are often accustomed to being in a reactive or retrospective mode. This is, in part, because it is often how they have been taught to manage their blood glucose. People will be less likely to operate in this reactive mode if they understand the importance and methodology of proactive bolus doses based on careful estimation of the carbohydrate they consume.

Correct for hyperglycemia prior to food intake

Use the correction factor for that time of day and/or for the level of blood glucose (smart pumps have the technology to set different CFs for different time periods of the day and/or for different blood glucose levels) to calculate and give a dose of rapid-acting insulin to begin to lower blood glucose prior to food intake. Research with lispro in hyperglycemic patients (blood glucose at start of meal 171–189 mg/dl) demonstrated that taking lispro 15 to 30 minutes before food consumption was ideal with hyperglycemia (Rassam et al. 1999). Another suggestion is that longer (>15 minutes) lag times are more desirable when there is more profound preprandial hyperglycemia (Mudaliar et al. 1999). Encourage people, if possible, to wait until the insulin begins to lower blood glucose before they eat in order to prevent an even greater rise of blood glucose and more difficulty lowering it. For example, if the blood glucose level is between 140 mg/dl and 180 mg/dl before the meal, administer rapid-acting insulin and wait 15–30 minutes before eating. If blood glucose is higher, waiting 30–45 minutes may be optimal. If these guidelines can't be used due to hunger or the need to eat at a particular time, advise the person to eat minimal carbohydrate (<15–30 grams) at the meal by choosing more nonstarchy vegetables and sources of protein. Another strategy is to check blood glucose 30–45 minutes before the meal. If blood glucose is high at this time, take a correction dose based on the CF. It's also worth noting that some people may delay, skip, or eat less at a meal if blood glucose levels are elevated, due to the lack of appetite caused by hyperglycemia.

Caveats

When using the above practical tips for managing preprandial hyperglycemia, teach the following caveats:

1. If a bolus dose is delayed, the entire action curve of that dose is delayed. This action curve (insulin on board) must be accounted for when deciding on the next bolus dose.

2. Don't get into the habit of skipping meals to manage hyperglycemia. These are tips to manage occasional hyperglycemia. Skipping meals frequently can put a person at risk for insufficient nutrient intake.

3. Always carry a source of carbohydrate to manage hypoglycemia if blood glucose decreases more quickly than expected or if food intake is delayed beyond the anticipated time.

4. For people who drive (and have the possibility of being delayed in traffic), operate machinery, or are in other situations where hypoglycemia could endanger themselves or others, these guidelines may not be safe to use.

Low blood glucose before a meal

If blood glucose is lower than desirable (<70 mg/dl) at mealtime, encourage people to take their insulin a few minutes after they start to eat rather than 10–15 minutes before the meal. This is especially important if they haven't treated the low blood glucose prior to eating; waiting to take their insulin allows the carbohydrate to start to raise the blood glucose level. This is particularly wise if the meal consists of foods that tend to take longer to raise blood glucose, such as high-fat or high-fiber foods.

One can also use the correction factor *in reverse*, administering less insulin to cover the meal. For example, if preprandial blood glucose is 60 mg/dl and the CF is 30 mg/dl, subtract one unit from the ICR-based bolus dose. However, if the person has treated the hypoglycemia and blood glucose is above 90 mg/dl at the point they begin to eat, they can feel comfortable taking their insulin before the start of the meal. Insulin pumps can, if set up to do so, apply a reverse correction to determine bolus doses.

Uncertain carbohydrate intake

If the amount of carbohydrate that will be consumed at a meal is uncertain, encourage people to split their dose of rapid-acting insulin as follows:

Take enough insulin 10–15 minutes before the meal to cover an amount of carbohydrate they know they will eat (i.e., 30–45 grams), as well as to cover an elevated blood glucose level, if necessary. People can then take the remainder of their bolus dose to cover the remaining carbohydrate they have consumed or will consume in the middle or at the end of the meal. This technique may also work well for meals that are larger than normal, as large meals can delay the rise of blood glucose regardless of their nutrient composition.

Longer or larger than usual meals

On occasion, people have meals that span more time than usual. It might be a holiday meal, a special occasion, or a lengthy dinner or cocktail party. Follow the same principles as when carbohydrate intake is uncertain.

Covering the carbohydrate in snacks

With rapid-acting insulin regimens, people no longer need to snack to prevent hypoglycemia between meals as they did with older insulins and regimens. There are several reasons for this, but primarily this is because rapid-acting insulin works more in sync with meals (if timed correctly) and long-acting insulin (glargine or detemir), if the dose is set correctly, causes less hypoglycemia because it is ostensibly peakless.

However, some people may still want to snack, and people in some age groups (i.e., preschoolers, school-aged children, and pregnant women) may need to snack to achieve adequate nutrition. People who snack need to be encouraged to take rapid-acting insulin to cover snacks if the food contains more than about 10 grams of carbohydrate. If insulin is not taken to cover this carbohydrate, blood glucose will rise and will need to be treated after the fact. People need to understand that a mere 10–15 grams of carbohydrate can raise blood glucose upwards of 30–50 mg/dl. People should be cautioned, however, that insulin taken to cover snacks between meals needs to be considered (insulin on board) when they take their next bolus. This will prevent insulin stacking.

*   *   *   *   *

Advising people about the use of rapid-acting insulin to achieve both lifestyle flexibility and optimal blood glucose control is challenging. This is due in part to the intricacies and variation of daily life as well as to the inter- and intra-individual variations in insulin action. With a greater understanding of the pharmacodynamic action of rapid-acting insulin and practical tips, people with diabetes can achieve and maintain improved blood glucose control more easily.

CHAPTER SEVEN

Advanced Carbohydrate Counting and Continuous Subcutaneous Insulin Infusion

There exists ample evidence that using continuous subcutaneous insulin infusion (CSII), or insulin pump, therapy to establish and maintain near normoglycemia can improve health and reduce the development of long-term diabetes complications (DCCT 1993; Pickup and Kenn 2002). A key factor in successful CSII therapy, however, is carbohydrate counting. It is absolutely essential that a person (or caretaker(s) if the person is a child or adult who needs assistance) learn and use Advanced Carbohydrate Counting skills for several weeks or months before beginning CSII therapy. Further, *it is both the prescribing clinician's, as well as the potential pump user's, responsibility that the prospective pumper has proficiency in Advanced Carbohydrate Counting.* Mastery of advanced carbohydrate skills requires education provided by an experienced diabetes educator, preferably a registered dietitian (RD), certified diabetes educator (CDE).

A person's knowledge of carbohydrate counting and their comfort level with adjusting prandial bolus insulin doses will provide a foundation for successful CSII therapy. Many clinicians and prospective pumpers alike do not realize that this is the responsibility of the pump prescriber and pumper/parent(s). Teaching Advanced Carbohydrate Counting skills is not the responsibility of a per diem pump trainer or pump manufacturer employee (i.e., sales representative, territory manager, clinical education specialist, clinical manager, etc.) on the day of the pump therapy training or initiation. At this point, it is too late in the process to begin teaching carbohydrate-counting methods and concepts. Ideally, a prospective pumper should be able to demonstrate Advanced Carbohydrate Counting skills several weeks (or months) before beginning CSII therapy.

There are countless stories of "pump therapy failures" or people whose pump therapy "just didn't work right." Many of these disheartening tales of failed CSII therapy can be traced to lack of knowledge of carbohydrate counting skills coupled with inaccurate basal doses, or, worse yet, lack of adjustment of basal rates with basal testing over time. There are even cases of people using an insulin pump with a set bolus dose per meal without any regard to the amount of carbohydrate to be consumed. *Again, Advanced Carbohydrate Counting mastery is a must for successful pump therapy.*

Several of the latest generation of insulin pumps assist in CSII therapy through use of an incorporated food database. Some are static, in that they simply provide carbohydrate counts of commonly eaten foods; others allow people to add the nutrition information for foods they commonly eat and then use this information to help calculate bolus doses. Some pumps also allow the user to build a personalized food database of commonly eaten favorite foods and beverages and then program these as preset amounts with user-assigned names, such as "cold cereal breakfast" or "lunch salad." Another innovative pump option enables the user to simply input meal items for dosing; the pump adds the carbohydrate grams, and based on personalized information programmed by the user, the pump calculates the appropriate carbohydrate bolus. Even with these advances in pump technology, it is essential that the user understand how to use insulin-to-carbohydrate ratios (ICR) and demonstrate their accurate and consistent use over time.

THE NUTS AND BOLTS: BASAL RATES AND BOLUS OPTIONS

Insulin pumps

Though insulin pumps all operate in generally the same manner—delivering insulin subcutaneously from a reservoir by means of a catheter or needle placed under the skin—insulin pumps vary widely in design and functions. The pump can be a disposable unit programmed by remote control, or a small device that contains a plastic disposable insulin cartridge or reservoir filled with rapid- or short-acting insulin and programmed by pushing buttons in specific sequences. Pumps can hold from about 200 units up to 315 units of insulin, but this varies based on the model and manufacturer.

Most pumps weigh less than 4 ounces and are no larger than the size of a cell phone. All insulin pumps are worn 24/7. Most connect to the person with a thin plastic infusion set (ranging from 23 inches to 43 inches) that have adhesive tape on the end to stick to the skin. A disposable pump is smaller, weighs less than a traditional pump, and is connected directly to the person via a self-stick infusion set without any tubing. This system uses a handheld device to direct the action of the pump through radio frequency.

Is the Patient Ready?

There are many criteria to assess a person's readiness for CSII therapy. It is not the intent here to provide a detailed guide to CSII initiation. For specifics about initiation and follow-up, refer to these American Diabetes Association publications: *Putting Your Patients on the Pump* (Bolderman 2002) and *Smart Pumping* (Wolpert 2002). Additional insulin pump therapy resources are also provided in Appendix I.

However, there are some general indicators of readiness. A prospective CSII candidate should be adept at answering the following questions related to carbohydrate counting and CSII therapy without hesitation:

1. Do you know which foods contain carbohydrate?
2. How do you know how much carbohydrate you eat (i.e., how do you count carbohydrate)?
3. How do you determine your preprandial insulin doses?
4. What is (are) your ICR(s)?
5. Do you know how long your insulin dose(s) lasts?
6. How do you treat hyperglycemia?
7. What is your correction factor (CF)?
8. How do you treat hypoglycemia?

Basal rates

As opposed to multiple daily injection (MDI) therapy, which generally utilizes intermediate- or long-acting insulins to provide basal, or background, insulin, CSII uses only rapid-acting or regular insulin. Basal levels are achieved through the constant delivery of programmed incremental doses during a 24-hour period. The insulin is delivered in small increments, ranging from 0.25 (or less with a programmed temporary rate) units/hour to several units/hour.

Basal rates can be set for different amounts at different times of the day, depending on the user's individual needs. People who have a dawn phenomenon, for example, may find that setting a higher basal rate from about 3 AM to 7 AM works well to control this rise in blood glucose. Also, a person's basal rate requirements can differ day-to-day, depending on hormonal changes (e.g., stages of a menstrual cycle), illness, stress, physical activity, and work schedules. Today's pumps can hold several different (four to seven, depending on the model) 24-hour basal rate profiles to accommodate lifestyle and physiologic needs. Pumps can also be programmed to temporarily increase or decrease the hourly basal rate based on unscheduled events, such as exercise, illness, alcohol consumption, or stress. Some clinicians and pumpers find that using an increased temporary basal rate for a few hours when consuming a high-protein, high-fat, or lengthy meal

Examples of basal rates (in units per hour)

Weekday pattern (limited physical activity):
- 12 AM–3 AM: 0.5
- 3 AM–8 AM: 0.7
- 8 AM–5 PM: 0.6
- 5 PM–12 AM: 0.5

Weekend pattern (increased physical activity for two consecutive days):
- 12 AM–3 AM: 0.35
- 3 AM–8 AM: 0.55
- 8 AM–5 PM: 0.45
- 5 PM–12 AM: 0.35

Use of temporary basal rate for stress using weekday pattern:
- 12 AM–3 AM: 0.5
- 3 AM–8 AM: 0.7
- 8 AM–5 PM: 0.6
- 2 PM–4 PM: (Temporary increase of 30% for job-related stress) 0.6 × 130% for 2 hours = basal rate of 0.78 units/hour for this period; pump automatically configures correct rate based on user's programming of +30% and automatically resumes preset basal rate of 0.6 units/hour at 4 PM for continuation to 5 PM.
- 5 PM–12 AM: 0.5

is also an effective strategy to achieve target glucose levels. Trial-and-error and record keeping can help determine what works best. For additional guidelines, refer to Appendix I.

Basal rates that are correctly determined allow the pump user to delay or skip meals, have more flexibility with meal choices, and sleep later than their usual wake-up time without adversely affecting their most recent glucose level. Ideally, when basal rates are properly configured, a person's glucose levels do not fluctuate by more than 30 mg/dl during sleep or over a five-hour period when no food is eaten (Walsh and Roberts 2006). It is important to first establish and fine-tune a person's basal rates in order to determine that the insulin-to-carbohydrate ratio (ICR) used for bolus doses is correct. *If the basal rates are not accurate, ICR(s) and correction factors (CF) will not be accurate* (Bolderman 2002).

All too often, clinicians discover that pump users have not made any adjustments in their basal rates. This is particularly disturbing, considering that people go through many lifestyle changes over the course of time, particularly growing children and adolescents. Testing basal rates will uncover glucose fluctuations and the accuracy/inaccuracy of the basal rates. Basal rate testing may take several attempts of two to three days each, and should be done periodically (about once a year). Lifestyle changes (such as job and activity level changes), weight loss or gain of more than 5 pounds, growth spurts, pregnancy, perimenopause, menopause, and the onset of complications (e.g., gastroparesis) are examples of situations that warrant basal rate testing and adjustment. Guidelines for testing and changing basal rates are found in various pump therapy books well as in journal articles. As advances are made, the use of continuous glucose monitoring (CGM) will also assist in the determination of appropriate basal rates.

Bolus doses

Standard bolus doses

Ideally, the person who begins or is already using CSII is familiar with carbohydrate counting and is using an established ICR. If the basal rates have been tested to verify their accuracy, the person's ICR(s) should be appropriate, but may also require adjustment. The ICR is used to match bolus insulin to the amount of carbohydrate to be consumed. Bolus doses can be fine-tuned to deliver insulin according to the pump user's needs. A bolus can be delivered in its entirety immediately, split equally into two separate bolus doses delivered in determined time intervals, extended in entirety over time, or split unequally—a portion of the bolus delivered at once, and the remainder of the bolus delivered over a designated extended period of time.

Pump manufacturers have devised various names for their "all-at-once" bolus delivery option. Examples include "standard bolus," "normal bolus," "immediate bolus," "quick bolus," and "now bolus." For usual mixed meals containing about 50% carbohydrate, 20% protein, and 30% fat, an immediate bolus is generally appropriate as long as the bolus is delivered about 10–15 minutes prior to the meal. Also appropriate for an immediate bolus delivery are meals or snacks that are >50% carbohydrate.

Bolus options: Extended (square wave) and combination (dual wave)

Pump manufacturers provide several options for bolus delivery, in addition to the standard all-at-once bolus. Examples generally fall under two categories:

- Extended or square wave bolus, where the total amount of the bolus is delivered over a user-determined period of time
- Combination, multiwave, or dual wave bolus, where a portion of the bolus is delivered "up front," or immediately, and the remainder is delivered over time

Examples of Standard Bolus Doses (in units of insulin)

Mixed (lunch) meal:	g carb	g protein	g fat
2 slices rye bread	36	2	0
1 ounce turkey		7	5
1 ounce American cheese		7	5
2 leaves lettuce	0	0	0
1 teaspoon mayonnaise	0	0	5
¾-ounce bag pretzel rings	15	2	0
1 medium apple	23	0.5	0
12-ounce can diet cola	0	0	0
Totals:	**74 g**	**18.5 g**	**15 g**
Calories per gram	× 4	× 4	× 9
Total kcal (505):	296 kcal	74 kcal	135 kcal
Percentages of nutrients:	58%	15%	27%

ICR is 1:15
Meal bolus: 74 grams ÷ 15 = 4.9 units

Since this is a typical mixed meal, the bolus of 4.9 units would be delivered in its entirety at once prior to the meal.

Carbohydrate snack	**Nutrients**
1 large banana	~35 grams carbohydrate, 0.5 g protein
Percentage of nutrient(s):	100% carbohydrate (rounded)

ICR is 1:12
Snack bolus: 35 ÷ 12 = 2.9 units

Since fruit is a typical carbohydrate snack, the bolus of 2.9 units would be delivered in its entirety at once prior to the snack.

In all cases, the pump wearer, relying on trial-and-error, clinician guidelines, experiences, and shared information with other pumpers, determines the amount of the bolus to be delivered and the amount of time that works best.

Extending a bolus provides coverage for foods or situations that increase the blood glucose gradually. Meals that take longer to consume, such as a brunch, cocktail party, or holiday celebration, may require that the bolus dose of insulin be adjusted for time. Also, for meals or snacks that may be higher in protein and/ or fat, some pump users have found that "spreading the bolus out over time" yields better postprandial glucose levels two, four, and six hours later.

Although there exists little scientific data to support the delayed elevation of prandial glucose from protein and/or fat intake (ADA 2008b; Franz 2000; Franz, et al. 2002; Gannon et al. 2001), many using CSII anecdotally report that adjusting their meal/snack bolus for a higher-than-usual consumption of protein and/or fat results in closer-to-target glucose levels (Ahern et al. 1993; Bolderman 2002; Chase et al. 2002; Jones et al. 2005; King and Armstrong 2007; Walsh and Roberts 2006; Wolpert 2002). The practice of extending a bolus delivery is a trial-and-error process. This process may take several weeks or months to complete, requiring experiments of bolus time durations and amounts and fastidious record-keeping on the part of the user. CGM records provide adjunctive assistance in developing time durations (Jones et al. 2005).

In addition to high-protein and/or high-fat meals, other situations that may warrant the need to use an extended or combination bolus include:

- Gastroparesis (delayed digestive emptying)
- Some medications, such as some tricyclic antidepressants, some anti-emetics, opioids, and anticholinergics
- Pramlintide (SYMLIN, amylin analog)

Pump manufacturers provide a variety of extended bolus delivery choices. Options range from 0–100% of the bolus immediately with the remainder deliv-

Pramlintide and CSII

Those who inject preprandial pramlintide (per manufacturer's instructions) while using CSII or MDI therapy are advised to decrease their ICR(s), because less insulin is needed to cover the same amount of carbohydrate previously covered before their pramlintide regimen. This practice is supported by the manufacturer's recommendation to reduce mealtime insulin by 50% upon the initiation of pramlintide and titrate as needed to achieve desired target glucose levels (SYMLIN 2005).

Example:
Pre-pramlintide: ICR is 1:15
Pramlintide initiation: ICR is 1:30
After one-month pramlintide use: ICR is 1:20

It is anecdotally reported that some pump users who inject pramlintide find they achieve improved postprandial glucose levels with the use of an extended or combination bolus. However, not enough research or evidence is available to support this guideline. Many pumpers who inject pramlintide find that trial-and-error adjustments in their insulin doses and timing will help achieve desired target glucose levels.

ered in single digit percentages anytime from 15 minutes to 24 hours in 15-minute increments. As of this publication date, one pump manufacturer provides the user the ability, with external software and the pump's infrared (IR) port transfer, to personalize and name a bolus with a 0–100% portion to be delivered immediately and the remainder over time (e.g., pizza bolus 32% immediate, 68% over 5 hours, 15 minutes; dessert bolus 55% immediate, 45% over 3.5 hours; ethnic meal bolus 50% immediate, 50% over 4 hours, etc.). Pumps vary in their features and options, and manufacturers routinely develop and offer new options and improvements, so it is important for the clinician to be aware of the various models and features available since many can make matching carbohydrate and insulin easier and more accurate.

There are no published lists, charts, guidelines, pamphlets, articles, or books that can provide personalized or individualized bolus option amounts and time durations that are appropriate for each person. Every pump user is different

Examples of Bolus Doses (Extended and Combination)

Snack Bolus
One 2-ounce chocolate candy bar with 20 grams of carbohydrate, 1 gram of protein, and 9 grams of fat.
ICR is 1:10
Snack bolus: 2 units
Extended bolus option: 2 units over 60 minutes

In this example, the pump user determined that the high fat content of the snack affected his two-, three-, and four-hour postprandial blood glucose readings.

Pizza Bolus
Combination bolus option: 36% immediately, 64% over 5 hours, 15 minutes.

Precise bolus dose amount varies, based on the grams of carbohydrate from the size and number of pizza slices consumed, but the unique nature of pizza calls for an individualized extended dose.

Thanksgiving Meal
Nutrients in the meal are 85 grams of carbohydrate, 42 grams of protein, and 43 grams of fat.
ICR is 1:12
Meal bolus: 7 units
Combination bolus option: 3.5 units immediate bolus, 3.5 units extended over 2 hours, 45 minutes.

and people react differently to foods consumed. To best determine appropriate customized boluses, the user should keep the following records for review and analysis. These factors will assist in making changes for bolus percentages and time durations:

- Preprandial glucose level
- Time of most recent bolus from previous meal/snack or correction
- Amount of most recent bolus from previous meal/snack or correction
- Duration of insulin action time remaining from previous meal/snack or correction (insulin on board)
- Amount of carbohydrate to be consumed
- Amount of protein to be consumed
- Amount of fat to be consumed
- Amount of alcohol to be consumed
- Calculation of total bolus
- Type of bolus delivery: immediate, extended, or combination
- If extended bolus delivery, duration of time
- If combination bolus delivery, percentage of bolus delivered immediately and percentage of bolus delivered over time
- If combination bolus delivery, duration of time for extended portion of delivery
- One-, two-, three-, four-, and if appropriate, five- and six-hours postprandial glucose results

Bolus considerations

A "missed" (omitted or forgotten) bolus can be deleterious to a person's glucose level (Burdick et al. 2004). Some pumps offer the convenience of setting reminders/alarms to remind the user to take certain actions. One alarm option on some pumps is the missed meal bolus alert alarm that can remind a person to deliver a bolus if they haven't taken a bolus within a specific time segment (such as between 6 AM and 10 AM for breakfast). Many pump users find this to be extremely helpful, while others may tend to ignore the alarms (Chase et al. 2002).

It's also worth noting that boluses are not foolproof. While it is important to teach those on CSII to accurately calculate their carbohydrate consumption and bolus accordingly, there will be instances when "unexplained" glucose excursions or decreases occur. After basal rates have been checked, adjusted, and verified, and the clinician and/or pump user has factored in or accounted for the effects of hormone changes, stress, exercise, illness, and alcohol consumption, the ICR(s) may need to be adjusted. This is especially true when there are recurrent out-of-target glucose levels. Refer to chapter 8 for information on how to adjust ICR(s).

CORRECTION DOSES AND CSII

Multiple CFs

As outlined previously in chapter 6, a correction, or supplemental, insulin dose is rapid- or short-acting insulin taken to return an elevated blood glucose level to target level. This dose is based on an individualized CF. No matter which method may have been used to calculate a person's CF (see various methods in chapter 6), today's pumps offer the user the option of programming individualized CFs. Some pumps offer the option to program CFs based on time of day, while others offer the option based on glucose levels.

Some people may need a different insulin CF at different times of the day or month. Evening, for example, is a time when many people are more sensitive to insulin. If one unit of insulin lowers a person's glucose about 50 mg/dl during the day, a higher CF may be needed at night (e.g., one unit may lower the person's glucose level 70 mg/dl in the evening).

Multiple Correction Doses Based on Level of Hyperglycemia

Blood glucose in the 100–200 mg/dl range:
Target 3-hour postprandial glucose level: 120 mg/dl
Current glucose level: 187 mg/dl
Glucose above target: 67 mg/dl
CF: 60 mg/dl (1 unit decreases glucose approximately 60 mg/dl)
Correction dose: 1.1 units (67 ÷ 60 = 1.1)
3-hour postprandial reading: 125 mg/dl

Blood glucose in the >200 mg/dl range:
Target 3-hour postprandial glucose level: 120 mg/dl
Current glucose level: 253 mg/dl
Glucose above target: 133 mg/dl
CF: 42 mg/dl (1 unit decreases glucose approximately 42 mg/dl); this CF is 30% lower than normal CF of 60 mg/dl
Correction dose: 3.1 units (133 ÷ 42 = 3.16, round to 3.1 or 3.0 units)
3-hour postprandial reading: 125 mg/dl

Trial-and-error and detailed record-keeping will help provide data to determine a person's CF when glucose levels are above 200 mg/dl.

The higher the glucose level, the more resistant/less sensitive a person is to insulin. Thus, more insulin may be required to return glucose levels to the desired target range depending on the current glucose level. Many people find that their normal CF is appropriate when glucose levels are in the 100–200 mg/dl range, but when glucose levels exceed 200–240 mg/dl, it is not as effective. In that case, a person may need to decrease his or her CF by 20–30% to provide more insulin. Some of today's pumps offer the option for the user to program several different CFs, as well as several blood glucose targets and ICRs.

Correction bolus doses

When the preprandial blood glucose level is above target, it will be necessary to supplement a meal insulin bolus with a correction insulin bolus dose. This bolus dose will be calculated using the CF, current blood glucose level, target blood glucose level, and amount of insulin "on board" (i.e., amount of bolus insulin remaining from the most recent bolus).

Most pumps can calculate the amount of insulin on board and suggest a decreased correction bolus dose or no bolus dose at all. The factors that the pump automatically configures in its calculation are

- current blood glucose level,
- target blood glucose level,
- CF,
- duration of insulin action,
- amount of insulin remaining from the most recent bolus, and
- carbohydrate grams or meal bolus dose (some pumps).

All current smart pumps subtract insulin on board from the most recent correction bolus when the current blood glucose level is elevated. But all current pumps do not subtract on-board insulin from the most recent carbohydrate bolus. Some pumps subtract on-board insulin from the most recent carbohydrate bolus only if the blood glucose level is below target. One current pump model offers this as an on/off option. Since insulin pumps differ in how they calculate on-board insulin, it is best to be familiar with the various pump models and to be aware of the differences when teaching people about correction bolus doses.

Duration of insulin action and remaining bolus insulin

As is evident from the impact of on-board insulin, the duration of insulin action time should be considered when determining an appropriate bolus dose, either a meal/snack bolus or correction bolus, or a combination of both. Although the onset, peak, and duration of action times for currently available rapid-acting insulins (and short-acting insulins) are usually cited as being similar, there can be slight differences (Walsh et al. 2003). Likewise, how people respond to the onset, peak, and duration of insulin can differ from person to person and day to day. Clinicians need to keep this in mind when deciding which rapid-acting insulin to select for use in an insulin pump, and this, in turn, can affect the programming of the duration of insulin action setting.

Relying on numerous correction bolus doses in a day indicates blood glucose control is less than optimal. Basal rate(s) and carbohydrate boluses need to be adjusted (increased) when correction bolus doses are more than 8% of a person's TDD (Walsh and Roberts 2006). Many factors, as discussed, can affect the blood glucose level, but an important consideration often overlooked, or not given enough attention, is the "insulin on board" remaining from the most recent bolus. For more information on how this correlates to improved control and fewer correction boluses, refer to chapter 8.

The "smart pumps" of today offer the ability to help people prevent insulin stacking with the insulin-on-board feature (if a person chooses to use it). The pumps use appropriate models of rapid-acting insulin action curves in their software to determine how much active insulin is still present in a person's body. The pump user has the option of choosing different time durations for the activity of their rapid-acting insulin. The prescribing clinician should discuss this option with the pump user *before* the person is to be trained on the pump. The duration of insulin action has a profound influence on the use and efficacy of correction boluses. Generally, a duration of 3–4 hours works for most people, but *the decision to program an appropriate insulin duration setting should be based on sound clinical judgment and should not be left to the discretion of a per diem or an industry pump trainer on the day of pump initiation/training.*

Factors to consider in programming an insulin pump for the "duration of insulin action" feature:

- Pump user's knowledge of and experience with
  - "how long my insulin lasts;"
  - recurrent postprandial hyperglycemia or recurrent hypoglycemia;
  - and the "vicious cycle" of the overtreatment of hyperglycemia resulting in hypoglycemia and/or overtreatment of hypoglycemia resulting in hyperglycemia.

- Clinician's knowledge of and experience with
  - using insulin action curves in advising a person about the "wait time" to administer a correction dose of insulin;
  - the person's specific insulin requirements, including previous insulin doses, sensitivity to insulin, recurrent hyper- and hypoglycemia, and,

if present, knowledge of the person's episodes of the "vicious cycle" of hyperglycemia overtreatment and hypoglycemia overtreatment;
- using insulin pump action curves and duration of insulin-on-board features.

To better understand how to advise a person about accurate correction bolus doses of insulin, it's important for the clinician to have an understanding of the pharmacokinetics versus pharmacodynamics of rapid-acting insulin. Refer to chapter 8 for information on this topic.

USEFUL PUMP FEATURES

When pumps were first introduced in the 1970s, and up until 2002, bolus doses were calculated by units of insulin manually input by the user. In 2002, with the introduction of the first "smart" pump by a newcomer (Smiths Medical/Deltec) to the insulin pump industry, it became possible for the pump to automatically calculate the units of insulin based on the total grams of carbohydrate programmed into the pump by the pump user. The pump would then suggest a bolus dose based on the user's individualized ICR. Soon after this concept was introduced, other pump manufacturers followed suit.

With many of today's pumps, the user selects the preferred method for the pump to calculate bolus doses. If using carbohydrate grams as the basis for bolus doses, the pump calculates a suggested meal bolus based on factors such as the amount of carbohydrate to be consumed, ICR, current glucose level, target glucose level, and amount of insulin remaining from a previous bolus. If using units of insulin as the basis for bolus doses, the user manually calculates the carbohydrate gram coverage and inputs the total number of insulin units to cover the carbohydrate into the pump. The pump can then confirm the dose or suggest a different dose based on other factors, including blood glucose level, target blood glucose level, and duration of insulin action from the most recent bolus.

In addition to bolus options and the availability to program individualized ICRs and CFs, some pumps also offer built-in carbohydrate count databases and/or the ability to personalize and build a customized carbohydrate count database. A carbohydrate count database may be programmed into the actual pump, its remote control device, or a personal digital assistant (PDA) device. A personalized carbohydrate database puts the information literally into the hands of the pump user when needed. Many people find this to be a helpful tool that alleviates the need to memorize carbohydrate counts of their favorite foods and beverages. A caution here is that the portion size listed in the database may not correspond to the person's actual serving size, so a mathematical calculation may be necessary.

Chapter 13 presents a process to help people develop their own customized database of carbohydrate counts.

As technology improves, pumps will continue to get "smarter," adding new features and improving the ease and accuracy of glucose control. Many available pumps are already equipped with advanced features and can:

- **Calculate a suggested amount of carbohydrate needed to return a low glucose level to target (reverse correction).** The user programs his/her current glucose level and the pump uses various factors, including on-board insulin, to suggest an appropriate amount of carbohydrate for the pump user to consume. This helps reduce the risk of overcorrecting hypoglycemia, preventing later hyperglycemia.
- **Provide averages of carbohydrate grams consumed by meal and/or by day and the amount of the carbohydrate bolus.** This helps the user and clinician track trends and make adjustments to ICRs as well as to overall dietary intake.
- **Total the amount of correction bolus insulin and provide correction bolus total percentages of the TDD.** This can aid the user/clinician in pattern management and help determine and change basal rates as well as ICRs and CFs.
- **Provide blood glucose readings and averages by meal or time.** Blood glucose values can be entered automatically by a meter attached to the pump, manually by the pump user, through radio frequency, or by infrared technology. Tracking blood glucose results can help to identify patterns and trends for making changes in basal rates, ICRs, CFs, bolus doses, and duration of insulin action times.
- **Give high and low blood glucose alerts as a reminder to take appropriate action.** Example: if the person has a "low" alert, this would indicate the need for hypoglycemia treatment.
- **Remind people when to check their blood glucose by setting alarms with personalized messages, such as "time to check blood glucose."**
- **Remind people of other factors that can affect their diabetes management, such as "take pills before dinner."**
- **Be programmed with other customized reminders, such as site change reminder, missed bolus reminder, time to check blood glucose reminder.**
- **Provide data that can be downloaded and stored, printed, or emailed.** The data can be for a time period of several months, such as 90 days/4000 events, and can include a history of TDD of insulin, meal boluses, correction boluses, basal rate profiles, basal rate changes, blood glucose results, alerts, and technical information, such as alarm history.

There are many pump models available, and both the clinician and the potential pump user must decide which model offers features that are best matched to the needs of the person. No matter which pump model is selected, people who choose CSII therapy must have knowledge of and experience with Advanced Carbohydrate Counting skills, including use of ICRs and CFs.

CHAPTER EIGHT

Pattern Management for Glycemic Control

Diabetes self-management encompasses solving problems and making decisions based on the ability to detect patterns in blood glucose and make proactive changes in the diabetes management plan, which includes medication, food, and physical activity. Knowing what, when, and how to make changes are the essence of successful diabetes self-management. Most importantly, every person should work with their health care provider to discuss and determine realistic blood glucose target levels. Targets should include fasting, preprandial, postprandial (one to two hours after the start of the meal), bedtime, and, if appropriate, during sleep. People with diabetes, and clinicians alike, cannot be expected to recognize "highs and lows" and glucose trends without knowing or establishing expected individualized target glucose levels.

PATTERN MANAGEMENT: THE KEY TO FINE-TUNING CONTROL

Pattern management is a comprehensive approach to blood glucose control that includes all aspects of current diabetes therapy (Hinnen et al. 2003). It involves reviewing several days of glucose records and making proactive adjustments based on trends, rather than reacting to a single high or low blood glucose reading (Hirsch and Hirsch 2001). Recognizing patterns in glucose control can assist both the clinician and the person with diabetes to identify factors that affect self-monitoring blood glucose (SMBG) results and make appropriate changes. In regard to Advanced Carbohydrate Counting, pattern management is essential in reviewing the efficacy of basal rates, insulin-to-carbohydrate ratios (ICR), and correction factors (CF) and making the proper adjustments.

Although pattern management is typically identified with intensive diabetes therapy, this approach should also include changes in combinations of oral agents to improve glycemic control as well as nonpharmacologic therapies, e.g., nutrition therapy and physical activity (Hinnen and Guthrie 2005). A review of the SMBG results should be done on a periodic and routine basis.

Pattern management involves reviewing several days of records and noting trends. Encourage people to record their information so that glucose values that occur at the same time each day can be seen as such and reviewed together. Many clinicians provide or suggest a form or booklet for the person to record pattern management information. These forms can either be assembled by the patient or clinician, or come preprinted from manufacturers or publishers. Glucose meters, insulin pumps, software programs, or web-based software programs also provide technology for capturing and downloading data. Continuous glucose monitoring (CGM) is another tool for tracking blood glucose results.

What to record

Encourage people to record as much information as they can. Pattern management is most effective when there exists a record of the following:

- **Medication:** diabetes (insulin, other injectables, oral agents) and non-diabetes medications that can affect blood glucose—names, doses, times, omissions
- **Glucose:** a minimum of three to four daily SMBG checks with times for three to four days/week—fasting, preprandial, postprandial (2 hours after the start of a meal), bedtime, and 3 AM readings, if appropriate; ideally, four to six daily SMBG results (or data from CGM) would be recorded to provide more information for detecting trends
- **Food:** including alcohol and other beverages; quantity and time consumed; specific carbohydrate amounts; missed meals or snacks
- **Physical activity:** planned or unplanned; time of day, duration, level of intensity
- **Treatment for hypoglycemia:** type and amount, e.g., amount of carbohydrate
- **Other factors:** travel, illness, stress, menses, insulin pump infusion set change, glucose sensor change, schedule changes, etc.; any event or occurrence that could affect blood glucose

Teach the person that it is necessary to record detailed information for a "complete picture." Although glucose meters, insulin pumps, and CGM devices capture glucose results and may also provide opportunity for the user to input additional information, devices usually cannot record personal detailed histories. Additionally, when people write down or record their information for themselves, they are more likely to take note and think about the causative factors for their blood glucose values.

To determine patterns, medication timing and doses, food intake, and activity levels must be as consistent as possible. This will help minimize blood glucose fluctuations that might otherwise mask true patterns. Changes in daily routines should also be noted along with other factors that can affect blood glucose.

Identify trends

Identify blood glucose trends in relation to the person's glucose target levels. Review blood glucose readings for the same time of day over several days of records. As a rule, three or more similar glucose values at the same time each day denote a trend. Several high readings at the same time of day is a trend. Several low readings at the same time of day is a trend. A trend becomes a pattern, and there can be multiple patterns in several days of records.

Before making assumptions on emerging patterns, however, make sure you have enough data with which to work.

- Are there enough readings representing different times of the day?
- Do the blood glucose readings reflect the peak action times of the insulin(s), and/or other injectable or oral diabetes medications? Blood glucose check times should include fasting, pre- and postprandial, bedtime, during sleep (for evaluating peak times of some medications), and between-meal times.
- Are foods and beverages recorded accurately? For example, a sandwich with two slices of bread contains less carbohydrate than a "club" sandwich or small sub sandwich.
- Is there a pattern(s) when evaluating three to five days of blood glucose readings?
- Does something happen at the same time every day, such as an insulin reaction, a high reading before the evening meal, etc.?
- What other factors that can affect glucose results are noted? Examples include exercise, illness, stress, infusion site/set changes, delayed or omitted medication doses, schedule changes, or overtreatment of hypoglycemia.
- Have there been changes in weight—loss or gain? Is there a recurrent pattern of weight change?

Once a pattern emerges

First, make sure glucose targets are established and understood. Several approaches to achieve target glucose levels exist. The "fix the fasting" method changes the basal insulin to normalize the fasting level without causing hypoglycemia during sleep. Another method is to conduct basal "check tests," where meals are delayed or omitted and other factors that can affect glucose (exercise, stress, alcohol, etc.) are eliminated for a minimum of four hours. Blood glucose levels are checked often and patterns noted.

Once glucose targets are established, adjust insulin to achieve target glucose levels with care to avoid hyperglycemia and hypoglycemia. Dose adjustments should not exceed one to two units and should be made only when a pattern of out-of-range glucose has been identified. Ideally, adjustments upward should be made every two to three days for rapid- or short-acting insulin, and every three to five days for intermediate- or long-acting insulin. Downward adjustments should be made the next day for unexplained hypoglycemia, especially if severe (Bode, ed. 2004). See Table 8-1 and Table 8-2 for specific adjustment options.

ADJUSTING THE ICR

Much information can be learned from detailed record keeping in pattern management. After reviewing records, noticing patterns and trends, and accounting for extenuating factors that may be contributing to trends, it may be necessary to adjust a self-management regimen. The following observations indicate the need for a change:

- Two to three daily correction boluses, or correction boluses that total about 8% of the total daily dose (Walsh and Roberts 2006)
- A correction bolus at the same time over a period of several days
- Consistent preprandial or two- to three-hour postprandial blood glucose above target level
- Consistent preprandial or two- to three-hour postprandial blood glucose below target level

Once the basal dose(s) of insulin(s) have been determined and verified to be appropriate, the ICR may need to be adjusted. The preferred method of adjusting ICR is similar to the preferred method of determining the initial ICR: using the personal information gathered through detailed SMBG record keeping.

Table 8-1. Possible Causes of Hyperglycemia and Adjustment Options

Possible Cause	Adjustment Options
Insufficient insulin to cover carbohydrate	Inaccurate carbohydrate counting (e.g., mixers in alcoholic beverages, breading on meat, poultry, fish, etc.); review carbohydrate calculations. The ICR may be too low; consider increasing the ICR. Example: use one unit of insulin to cover less carbohydrate, e.g., 1:12 instead of 1:15. Bolus may have been missed. If using continuous subcutaneous insulin infusion (CSII), set missed meal bolus alerts/alarms to prevent omission of bolus dose(s).
Excessive intake of protein and/or fat	Increase dose(s) of basal insulin. Consider splitting the bolus dose—a portion at beginning of meal and remainder 1/2 to 1 hour later. If using CSII, consider use of extended or combination bolus feature OR increased temporary basal rate(s).
Insufficient basal insulin	Increase basal dose(s) of insulin. If fasting, review time of most recent basal dose. Example: 24-hour basal dose no longer effective due to sleeping later on weekend or day off. If using CSII, this will occur only when basal rate(s) are inaccurate.
Insulin timing not matched to meal intake	Review timing of insulin dose (see chapter 12).
Medication dose not timed to meal intake	Review timing of medications such as pramlintide, alpha-glucosidase inhibitors, and meglitinides (see chapter 12).

Table 8-1. Possible Causes of Hyperglycemia and Adjustment Options *(cont.)*

Insulin dose not timed to account for delayed digestion (gastroparesis)	Delay rapid-acting insulin until during or after meal. Consider switching from rapid-acting to short-acting (regular) insulin. Discuss potential use of GI motility medications. If using CSII, consider use of extended or combination bolus feature OR decreased/increased temporary basal rate(s).
Insulin dose or diabetes medication dose unclear or omitted	Provide strategies to remember to take meds, such as alarms, notes, etc. If using CSII, set bolus dose reminders/alerts.
Inaccurate CF	Use lower CF. Example: one unit lowers glucose 40 mg/dl instead of 50 mg/dl.
Too much time between correction bolus doses	Review duration of insulin action time. Decrease time between bolus correction doses. If using CSII, adjust and follow insulin-on-board/duration of insulin action settings and reminders.
Overtreatment of hypoglycemia	Review "Rule of 15": consume 15 grams of carbohydrate and check blood glucose in 15 minutes; if not at target, repeat treatment until blood glucose reaches target. Review appropriate treatment for hypoglycemia: type and amount of carbohydrate. If using CSII, use correction bolus feature (for reverse recommendation).
Decrease in usual exercise or physical activity	Increase ICR(s). Example: use one unit of insulin to cover less carbohydrate, e.g., 1:12 instead of 1:15. Consider changing basal insulin dose; increase basal dose on days with less exercise. If using CSII, use temporary increased basal rate for several hours or alternate non–exercise day basal profile.

Table 8-1. Possible Causes of Hyperglycemia and Adjustment Options *(cont.)*

Initiation of new medication or dosage change	Review and confirm correct dose(s).
	Review blood glucose effects of new medications, e.g., addition of glucocorticoid.
	Increase ICR(s) and/or decrease CF(s). Example: use one unit of insulin to cover less carbohydrate, e.g., 1:12 instead of 1:15. OR, using a lower CF, 1 unit of insulin lowers glucose 40 mg/dl instead of 50 mg/dl.
Onset of illness; dental surgery; other surgeries	Notify health care provider.
	Check ketones (especially with type 1 diabetes).
	Increase non-caloric fluids if appropriate.
	Increase diabetes medication doses.
	Increase ICR(s) and/or decrease CF(s). Example: use one unit of insulin to cover less carbohydrate, e.g., 1:12 instead of 1:15. OR, using a lower CF, 1 unit of insulin lowers glucose 40 mg/dl instead of 50 mg/dl.
	If using CSII, implement increased temporary basal rates.
Emotional stress	Review intake: eating more than usual?
	Increase diabetes medication doses.
	Increase ICR(s) and/or decrease CF(s). Example: use one unit of insulin to cover less carbohydrate, e.g., 1:12 instead of 1:15. OR, using a lower CF, 1 unit of insulin lowers glucose 40 mg/dl instead of 50 mg/dl.
	If using CSII, consider alternate higher basal rates or temporary increased basal rates.
Menses/hormonal changes	Increase diabetes medication doses.
	Increase ICR(s) and/or decrease CF(s). Example: use one unit of insulin to cover less carbohydrate, e.g., 1:12 instead of 1:15. OR, using a lower CF, 1 unit of insulin lowers glucose 40 mg/dl instead of 50 mg/dl.
	If using CSII, consider alternate higher basal rates or temporary increased basal rates.

Table 8-1. Possible Causes of Hyperglycemia and Adjustment Options *(cont.)*

	If Using CSII
May be using incorrect basal rates (24-hour or temporary), target glucose level(s), ICRS(s), CF(s), or duration of insulin action/on-board insulin	Review pump time/date selection, basal rate selection/ programming (24-hour or temporary), target glucose level(s), ICRS(s), CF(s), and duration-of-insulin-action (insulin-on-board) settings. If incorrect, recalculate.
Batteries may be dead; alarm ignored or not heard/felt	Replace batteries.
Insulin cartridge/ reservoir empty	Replace cartridge/reservoir. Verify insulin has not expired.
Tubing may be occluded, contain air, become dislodged, or have cracks	Replace tubing/infusion set or replace pod.
Infusion site red, irritated due to infection, or set not changed within two to three days or according to schedule	Change site and infusion set or pod more frequently. Use pump site/set change reminder alarm.

Notes:
- It's best to fine-tune insulin doses related to carbohydrate first before making other insulin dose changes.
- Always try one method at a time.
- Planned exercise does not guarantee a decrease in hyperglycemia. People with diabetes may experience hyperglycemia if they exercise while under-insulinized or with the presence of ketones.
- To correct preprandial hyperglycemia, people can be encouraged to take one or more immediate actions:
  1. Increase the amount of the preprandial insulin dose, based on the CF.
  2. Decrease the amount of carbohydrate at the meal, but do not increase the preprandial insulin dose. Base the amount of reduced carbohydrate on the CF—the person should know the amount of carbohydrate that will increase their blood glucose a certain number of mg/dl and then deduct the carbohydrate amount accordingly.
  3. If using CSII, use the pump setting that suggests an increased amount of insulin, i.e., an individualized appropriate correction dose based on the programmed CF and target glucose level.

Table 8-2. Possible Causes of Hypoglycemia and Adjustment Options

Possible Cause	Adjustment Options
Too much insulin to cover carbohydrate	Inaccurate carbohydrate counting; review carbohydrate calculations.
	If taking medications that promote satiety (e.g., pramlintide), preprandial carbohydrate estimate may be higher than actual carbohydrate ingested.
	The ICR may be too high; decrease the ICR. Example: use one unit of insulin to cover more carbohydrate, e.g., 1:15 instead of 1:12.
Decreased intake of protein and/or fat	Decrease dose(s) of basal insulin.
	If splitting bolus dose, reduce percentage of upfront bolus and increase percentage of remainder dose.
	If using CSII, recalculate duration of time and/or percentage of immediate and extended bolus duration.
Too much basal insulin	Decrease basal dose(s) of insulin.
Insulin timing not matched to meal intake	Review timing of insulin dose (see chapter 12).
Medication dose not timed to meal intake	Review timing of medications such as alpha-glucosidase inhibitors or meglitinides (see chapter 12).
Insulin dose not timed to account for delayed digestion (gastroparesis or gastric delay due to pramlintide)	Delay rapid-acting insulin until during or after meal.
	Consider switching from rapid-acting to short-acting (regular) insulin.
	Discuss potential use of GI motility medications.
	If using CSII, consider use of extended or combination bolus OR decreased/increased temporary basal rate(s).

Table 8-2. Possible Causes of Hypoglycemia and Adjustment Options *(cont.)*

Insulin dose or diabetes medication dose unclear	Review and confirm dose(s). Provide strategies to remember to take correct dose of meds, i.e., alarms, notes, etc.
Inaccurate CF	Use higher CF. Example: one unit lowers more blood glucose (50 mg/dl instead of 40 mg/dl)
Too many correction bolus doses, i.e., "stacking insulin"	Review timing of correction dose(s) and duration of insulin action. Increase time duration between bolus correction doses. If using CSII, adjust and follow duration of insulin action settings and reminders.
Increase in usual exercise or physical activity	Decrease ICR(s), e.g., 1:15 instead of 1:12 (1 unit covers more carbohydrate) Consider changing basal insulin dose; decrease basal dose on days with less exercise. If using CSII, use temporary decreased basal rate for several hours or alternate non–exercise day basal profile.
Initiation of new medication or dosage change	Review and confirm correct dose(s). Review blood glucose effects of new medications, e.g., ß-blockers.
Onset of illness; dental surgery; other surgeries	Notify health care provider. Check ketones (especially with type 1 diabetes). Substitute solid carbohydrate foods with liquid carbohydrate, if tolerated. May need to decrease ICR(s) and increase CF(s). Example: use one unit of insulin to cover less carbohydrate, e.g., 1:20 instead of 1:15. OR, using a higher CF, 1 unit of insulin lowers glucose 60 mg/dl instead of 50 mg/dl.

Table 8-2. Possible Causes of Hypoglycemia and Adjustment Options *(cont.)*

Emotional stress	Possibly decrease diabetes medication doses; decrease ICR(s) and increase CF(s), or if using CSII, consider alternate lower basal rates or temporary decreased basal rates.
Menses/hormonal changes	Decrease diabetes medication doses. Decrease ICR(s) and increase CF(s). If using CSII, consider alternate lower basal rates or temporary decreased basal rates.
Alcohol intake	Review alcohol intake: quantity, type. Remind people that alcohol can lower blood glucose for up to 12 hours. Increase frequency of SMBG the morning after alcohol consumption. Consider reducing next morning insulin dose(s) or consuming additional carbohydrate 6–12 hours after alcohol consumption.

If Using CSII

May be using incorrect basal rates (24-hour or temporary), target glucose level(s), ICR(s), CF(s), and duration-of-insulin-action/on-board insulin	Review pump time/date selection, basal rate selection/programming (24-hour or temporary), target glucose level(s), ICR(s), CF(s), and duration-of-insulin-action settings; if incorrect, recalculate.

Table 8-2. Possible Causes of Hypoglycemia and Adjustment Options *(cont.)*

May have incorrect placement of infusion set	Check site selection and review appropriate site selection to avoid intra-muscular placement.

Notes:
- It's best to fine-tune insulin doses related to carbohydrate first before making other insulin dose changes.
- Always try one method at a time.
- To correct preprandial hypoglycemia, people can be encouraged to take one or more immediate actions:
  1. Treat the hypoglycemia with an appropriate amount of carbohydrate. Base the amount of carbohydrate on the CF. Do not increase the preprandial bolus dose to cover the carbohydrate consumed for the treatment of the hypoglycemia. Clinicians often use the "Rule of 15": consume 15 grams of carbohydrate, check blood glucose. If not at target, repeat treatment until blood glucose reaches target. The caveat is that this general rule may be too much or not enough carbohydrate for some people.
  2. If using CSII, use the pump setting that suggests an individualized appropriate amount of carbohydrate to increase the blood glucose level. Do not increase the preprandial bolus dose.
  3. Increase the amount of carbohydrate at the meal, but do not increase the preprandial insulin dose. Base the amount of additional carbohydrate on the CF, i.e., the person should know the amount of carbohydrate that will increase their blood glucose a certain number of mg/dl and consume the amount of carbohydrate that will return levels to target. This method of treating hypoglycemia is best for people who are not concerned about weight gain, since the increased amount of carbohydrate adds calories. For those who are concerned with weight gain, reducing insulin is a better choice.
  4. If using CSII, use the pump setting that suggests a reduced amount of insulin for the preprandial bolus, i.e., an individualized appropriate correction dose based on the programmed CF and target glucose level.
  5. Delay the preprandial insulin dose until during or after the meal. This gives the food a chance to raise blood glucose. Check blood glucose 15–20 minutes after the beginning of the meal and give the meal insulin dose when glucose begins to rise.

Food diary, insulin bolus dose, and SMBG information

When considering an ICR adjustment, ask the person to keep at least two to three days of records, including:

- Fasting, preprandial, and two-hour (after the start of the meal) postprandial glucose results
- Amount of carbohydrate consumed at meals, snacks, and other times (e.g., for hypoglycemia treatment); it is helpful for people to eat the same amount

of carbohydrate for breakfasts, lunches, evening meals, and snacks for the week of keeping records
- ICR(s) used
- Bolus insulin doses
- Exercise, illness, stress, menses, and alcohol consumption, including times and other related details of these factors (such as duration and intensity of exercise, pre/onset/duration of menses, amount of alcohol, etc.)

An example of a useful, detailed record would contain information similar to this:

- Preprandial blood glucose within target range
- Consumed 66 grams of carbohydrate
- Used six units of bolus insulin (rapid- or short-acting)
- Two-hour postprandial glucose is within target range
- $66 \div 6 = 11$
- ICR is 1 unit of insulin to 11 grams of carbohydrate

Making adjustments

Based on the personal SMBG records, it may be necessary to make adjustments. Based on either recurring hyper- or hypoglycemia, make the following changes:

- If blood glucose is consistently above target levels, adjust the ICR upward so that one unit of insulin covers less carbohydrate (e.g., change ratio from 1:12 to 1:10).
- If blood glucose is consistently below target levels, adjust the ICR downward so that one unit covers more carbohydrate (e.g., change ratio from 1:12 to 1:14).

Avoid making drastic changes. Adjustments to ICR(s) should be made by two to five grams at a time and then readjusted if target glucose levels are still not reached. For example, if postprandial blood glucose is consistently elevated, increase a ratio of 1:12 to 1:10 and then continue record keeping. New ICRs should be used for several days before making additional adjustments. Keeping detailed records is critical.

USING FEWER CORRECTION BOLUSES

When pattern management reveals the use of two to three daily correction boluses or a correction bolus at the same time over a period of several days, it may be time to make an adjustment. Consider the following factors that affect insulin doses:

- Insulin basal dose(s)
- ICR(s)
- Insulin CF(s)

Once the basal insulin and ICR(s) have been determined, evaluated, and verified as appropriate, the CF may need to be adjusted. Based on either recurrent hypo- or hyperglycemia, make the following adjustments:

- If corrected blood glucose level is still above target, adjust the CF downward so that one unit reduces more glucose (e.g., CF of 50 mg/dl reveals blood glucose was reduced only 45 mg/dl; decrease correction factor to 45 mg/dl).
- If corrected blood glucose level ends up below target, adjust the CF upward so that one unit reduces less glucose (e.g., CF of 50 mg/dl reveals blood glucose fell below target and was reduced 60 mg/dl; increase CF to 60 mg/dl).

Much like changes to ICR(s), changes to CF(s) should be done gradually and in small increments of 5 mg/dl so as not to potentiate hyperglycemia and hypoglycemic occurrences.

Data interpretation

Careful SMBG and record-keeping will help to establish patterns for when and how to make adjustments. Teach people that they should check blood glucose values for a reason—i.e., "check smart" versus "check often." Throughout their life with diabetes, people have different needs and desires that affect how and when to adjust their daily regimens. The frequency of checking blood glucose levels, keeping records, and identifying the emergence of trends and patterns will vary.

Pramlintide and Exenatide: Making Adjustments

Pramlintide

When using pramlintide as an adjunct to insulin, there are a number of considerations that need to be made, especially in terms of adjusting insulin dosage. Pramlintide, approved for use with mealtime insulin, should be taken with meals or snacks containing at least 250 calories or 30 grams of carbohydrate. At the outset, prandial insulin should be reduced by 50%, meaning ICRs should be adjusted as well (e.g., an ICR of 1:10 should change to 1:20). This may lead to postprandial hyperglycemia in the beginning. During this initial period, detailed SMBG records should be recorded and used to adjust prandial insulin dosages according to the manufacturer's suggested regimen. It is recommended that during the pramlintide initiation period, people perform a minimum of six to eight SMBG checks per day—fasting, preprandial, two-hour postprandial, and bedtime—and keep in close contact with a health care professional who is skilled in insulin use and dose adjustment. Eventually, prandial insulin doses will probably be adjusted upward. As pramlintide promotes satiety and decreases food intake, some suggest, "Take pramlintide with the first bite (of food), insulin with the last." Many using CSII have found that an extended or combination bolus works well with pramlintide, though not enough research or evidence is available to recommend this guideline.

Exenatide

Exenatide's actions are glucose-dependent and injected without regard to caloric or carbohydrate intake. Initially, it's recommended to inject the starting dose of exenatide within 60 minutes of the morning and evening meals (or at least six hours between the two main meals of the day) and decrease any sulfonylurea dose to prevent hypoglycemia. In some cases, if a person is experiencing marked postprandial hyperglycemia, the clinician may choose to maintain the person's usual sulfonylurea dose and not reduce it with the initiation of exenatide. Advise people to be aware of the increased satiety effect of exenatide and the need to not "force feed" themselves. It may take time for a person to adapt to feeling satisfied with smaller portions. A review of appropriate portion sizes, healthy foods, and meal planning may be beneficial.

CHAPTER NINE

Advanced Carbohydrate Counting Case Studies

CASE STUDY #1: DAVE

Dave's story is continued from the case studies in chapter 5 (see page 45). He is a 59-year-old widower who has had type 2 diabetes for 16 years. His food habits and schedule remain the same.

Regimen:
- Before breakfast: 25 units of 75/25 (mix of 75% insulin lispro protamine suspension and 25% insulin lispro [rDNA origin]), 45 mg pioglitazone (Actos)
- Before evening meal: 20 units of 75/25 (mix of 75% insulin lispro protamine suspension and 25% insulin lispro [rDNA origin])

Action Plan
The following action plan was devised at Dave's individual counseling appointment.

1. **Change split-mixed insulin regimen to rapid-acting and long-acting insulin analog regimen. Explain rapid-acting and long-acting insulin analog onset, peak, duration, and choice of methods of delivery (pen and syringe/vial).**

   The dietitian introduced information about rapid-acting insulin analogs, explaining that the onset, peak action, and duration times could help Dave improve his postprandial glucose levels. She also explained how peakless insulin, given at bedtime, could help prevent Dave's postprandial hypoglycemia. The peakless insulin will work throughout the next day to manage Dave's glucose levels between meals. Dave was agreeable to switching to a separate injection of rapid-acting insulin before meals and long-acting peakless insulin at bedtime. Based on the information provided by the dietitian, Dave felt that using only the rapid-acting insulin would be a better match to his mealtimes and meal choices and the peakless insulin at night wouldn't cause those "low blood sugar insulin reactions" right before bedtime. Dave was initially wary of adding two more injections, but when the dietitian reminded him about the added flexibility with meal choices and portions, Dave expressed more interest and was receptive to the idea.

The dietitian also introduced the idea of using an insulin pen and provided Dave with a demonstration. Dave was willing to try the switch and take the extra injections, saying "The fingersticks hurt more than the insulin needle, so taking two more shots with a tiny needle is not really a big deal, especially if I can eat less and take less insulin to match what I want to eat." Dave also thought using a pen at his evening meal would be more convenient than carrying a syringe and vial of insulin to restaurants and his lady friend's house. He was unaware that he could have been using a pen for his 75/25 insulin injections and was glad to learn this information.

2. **Explain the rationale for using an insulin-to-carbohydrate ratio (ICR) and correction factor (CF).**

The dietitian determined Dave was ready to advance to learning about ICRs and CFs. She explained how using these formulas would provide more flexibility in meal choices and portions. Dave verbalized understanding and agreed that he would have more "freedom to eat more or eat less, and not worry about low blood sugar when eating less." Dave also realized he could correct hyperglycemia without compromising his meal choices. The dietitian also suggested Dave increase his self monitored blood glucose (SMBG) to include a fourth check at bedtime to get an idea of how his glucose numbers were running after his evening meal.

3. **Determine Dave's ICRs and CFs.**

Based on Dave's records, as well as The Rule of 500 as a double check, the dietitian and Dave determined his ICR would be one unit of insulin to 12 grams of carbohydrate (500 ÷ 45 = 11.11, rounded up to 12). They also determined his CF based on the 1500 Rule. At a current total daily dose (TDD) of insulin of 45 units, Dave's CF is about 35 mg/dl (1500 ÷ 45 = 33, rounded up to 35).

4. **Assess Dave's understanding and application of his ICR and CF.**

Using one day of Dave's food and SMBG records, Dave demonstrated his ability to use the formulas to determine how much insulin he would take before meals. Dave was also able to figure out a correction dose of insulin to add to his meal dose when necessary. He realized learning this was going to be time consuming at first, but also realized how it made sense. The dietitian also cautioned Dave about weight gain, since he hadn't made much progress losing weight in the past few months. She explained it might be tougher to lose weight with the added flexibility he was going to have, but Dave said he would try to be careful and would cut down on some of his portions, specifically French fries with his fast food meals and rolls at his evening meal.

5. **Schedule an appointment to teach Dave how to use insulin pen(s).**
   The dietitian suggested Dave practice using his ICR and CF for a week "on paper" and either fax or mail his records to her for review. She suggested Dave call or schedule an appointment with his nurse practitioner to obtain prescriptions for insulin lispro and insulin glargine. Dave and the dietitian scheduled an appointment for him to return in three to four weeks to learn how to use the disposable insulin pens and initiate using his insulin-to-carbohydrate ratio and correction factor.

Dave's Goals

The following goals were derived after discussing Dave's Action Plan at his last appointment.

1. **Add a fourth SMBG check to bedtime.**
   This will help Dave figure out if/when he needs to use a CF in the evening and also provide him with information on how his carbohydrate intake at dinner affects his bedtime glucose levels.

2. **Practice using his ICR on paper for a week and fax or mail his records to the dietitian.**
   By using his current blood glucose and food records to calculate preprandial insulin doses and correction doses, Dave will be able to assess how much carbohydrate he consumes and how his intake affects his blood glucose levels. He will also gain confidence in using his ratio and CF "on paper" before implementing with his new insulin regimen.

3. **Schedule an appointment with his nurse practitioner to obtain prescriptions for insulin lispro disposable pens and insulin glargine disposable pens.**
   Dave will obtain the necessary prescriptions for his new insulin regimen and then get his prescriptions filled for insulin lispro and insulin glargine disposable pens.

4. After obtaining his new disposable pens, return to meet with the dietitian to learn how to use the pens and initiate using his ICR and CF.

Follow-Up

1. Dave mailed eight days of records to the dietitian. His first few days of records indicated sporadic calculations with omissions at lunch and missing bedtime SMBG results. The remaining records were more complete and revealed good understanding of using his ICR and CF. The dietitian questioned the carbohydrate totals at three meals, noting that those meals were fast food. She marked his records accordingly. The dietitian also made notes about Dave's glucose results, with lunch fast food meals causing higher two-hour postprandial results in the high 200s.

2. The dietitian called Dave to review some of his records over the phone, noting the meal totals in question. Dave said he would pay more attention to how he added up the carbohydrate grams for fast food meals, and was trying to eat fewer fast food meals because he hadn't realized how much carbohydrate fast food meals contained. He said he was anxious to switch over to his new regimen and to learn how to use his pens. Dave and the dietitian set a date and time to meet in three weeks.

Dietitian's Action Plan

After the follow-up with Dave, the dietitian developed a quick action plan.

1. Teach Dave how to use his prescription lispro and glargine pens.

2. Review Dave's SMBG and food records with him.

The Next Appointment

Dave brought his disposable pens with the dosage prescription from his nurse practitioner to the appointment with the dietitian. His bedtime insulin glargine dose was 20 units and his Actos 45 mg dose was to be continued. The dietitian taught Dave how to use the disposable insulin pens and Dave demonstrated his understanding of the technique.

Dave and the dietitian then reviewed the records he had mailed. Dave also brought in recent records from the past three days and said he had cut down on fast food from four days a week to three days a week, with a goal of going down to two lunches a week. The dietitian reviewed his recent records and congratulated Dave on his improved calculations and intake of fewer fast food meals. Dave said he felt he understood how to use his ICR and CF and was ready to proceed with switching over to his new regimen. He agreed to keep detailed records for review in one to two weeks.

Dave and the dietitian set up a time to speak over the phone in three days to review his first few days using his new regimen. He had scheduled an appointment with his nurse practitioner for two months out and his return visit with the dietitian was set for three months.

Follow-Up

1. Dave called the dietitian in four days (late one day) and said he thought "things are going great." He thought his blood sugars looked better, and he had not yet had any hypoglycemia after his evening meal. He promised to mail the next few days' results to the dietitian.

2. Dave's mailed records indicated his 1:12 ICR and 35 mg/dl CF worked well most of the time. Upon review of his records, the dietitian noted on two occasions Dave had consumed additional carbohydrate at lunch (larger-sized sub rolls instead of his usual hamburger-sized rolls). His 2 1/2-hour postprandial glucose levels on those days were 278 mg/dl and 302 mg/dl. Dave had calculated his mid-afternoon CF insulin dose correctly, but still had out-of-target results three hours later.

3. The dietitian called Dave back to discuss his results. She commended Dave on his strong efforts and diligence in applying his new information and keeping detailed records. She also taught Dave that when his glucose exceeds 250 mg/dl, he becomes less sensitive to insulin and may need a lower CF (i.e., blood glucose >250 mg/dl does not decrease as much from one unit of insulin when compared with the decrease in blood glucose <250 mg/dl). Based on his results, the dietitian suggested he use a CF of 25 mg/dl when his blood glucose is >250 mg/dl. Dave verbalized understanding of the information, and said he would try that next time. The dietitian and Dave confirmed that his next appointment with her was in about 2 1/2 months, following his appointment with his nurse practitioner in about two months.

Dave's Action Plan

Based on the follow-up discussion, the following revised action plan was developed for Dave.

1. **Continue his new regimen.**
   - Insulin lispro before meals, based on his ICR of 1:12 with a CF of 35 mg/dl

when blood glucose <250 mg/dl and 25 mg/dl when blood glucose >250 mg/dl.

- 30 units of insulin glargine at bedtime
- Pioglitazone (Actos) 45 mg

2. **Call the dietitian if he has recurrent (three to five times/week) unexplained two- to three-hour postprandial glucose levels above or below his target levels.**

   If this is the case, Dave is aware he may need an additional review of carbohydrate counting with emphasis on portion control and/or adjustments in his ICR.

3. **Obtain blood work seven to ten days prior to his appointment with his nurse practitioner in two months.**

Follow-Up

Two months later at Dave's appointment with his nurse practitioner, Dave's A1C is down from 8.7% to 8.1%. His weight decreased 1 pound. Dave told his nurse practitioner he didn't mind the extra injections at lunch and bedtime because he was having fewer low blood sugar reactions and felt "more in control of my blood sugars than I was before." He also said "I got used to just figuring out how much insulin I needed to cover my carb, and I eat a lot of the same meals, so it's not a big deal. But when I want to eat more or less, that's when this is really great. I don't have to worry about having low blood sugars or going too high now that I control my own insulin."

Dave's nurse practitioner praised Dave for his hard work and advised him to continue his current regimen and return in four months.

Four months later, Dave reported his improved A1C result to the dietitian. He also said he found using his 1:12 ICR worked well when he was careful counting his carbohydrate accurately. He said as long as his blood sugars are <250 mg/dl, his CF of 35 mg/dl worked, but when he was >250 mg/dl, he changed his CF from the suggested 25 mg/dl to 20 mg/dl. Dave said he was having fewer occasions to use his lower CF, and he felt very comfortable using all his new information. He also said he really liked using the disposable insulin pens.

When the dietitian downloaded Dave's meter, she pointed out to Dave that he may need a higher ICR at breakfast, since his pre-lunch readings were higher than readings at other times of the day. She suggested he try a 1:10 ratio at breakfast, and keep lunch and dinner at 1:12. Dave verbalized understanding and said he would try this. A return appointment was set for 5 months.

CASE STUDY #2: BARBARA

History

Barbara is a 47-year-old married mother of two boys, aged 20 and 18. She has had type 1 diabetes for 23 years. Barbara works part-time 18–22 hours a week as a greeting card retail merchandiser supervisor. She has self-scheduled flexible daytime hours four days/week.

Data

Ht: 5′6″, Wt: 141 pounds, weight gradually increased 10 pounds in past five years. Preprandial target glucose level established by her physician: 100–150 mg/dl. A1C levels also gradually increased in past few years.

Regimen

Barbara's insulin regimen for the past six years has been a set dose of a rapid-acting insulin analog before each meal with a supplemental sliding scale for hyperglycemia and a bedtime dose of a long-acting insulin, recently switched to a long-acting insulin analog. Her physician has adjusted her doses yearly, and for the past year her doses have been:

- Insulin aspart:
  - Before breakfast: 7 units
  - Before lunch: 5 units
  - Before evening meal: 6 units
- Supplement with:
  - 101–150 mg/dl: 1 unit
  - 151–200 mg/dl: 2 units
  - 201–250 mg/dl: 3 units
  - 251–300 mg/dl: 5 units, check ketones
  - 301–351 mg/dl: 7 units, check ketones
  - 351–400 mg/dl: 9 units, check ketones
  - >400 mg/dl: 11 units, check ketones and call physician for additional instructions
- Insulin detemir: 24 units 9:30–10:00 PM.

Barbara uses a disposable insulin pen for her pre-lunch doses and a syringe and vial for her other injections.

Other medical conditions

- Retinopathy
- Mild controlled hypertension
- Mild recurrent adhesive capsulitis treated successfully with shoulder manipulation two years ago

Food habits/daily schedule

Workdays

- Wakes at 7:00 AM
- Breakfast: 7:30 AM—8 ounces orange juice, one bowl corn flakes or granola cereal, 8 ounces 2% milk, coffee with sugar substitute
- Lunch: Variable time between Noon to 1 PM—Packed sandwich from home, made of two slices turkey or ham or roast beef, one slice American or provolone cheese, and two slices rye or wheat bread; one small bag pretzels or chips; diet soda
- Evening meal: Between 5:30 and 6:30 PM—Tossed salad with 2 tablespoons regular dressing, 3–4 ounces meat, poultry, or fish (sometimes breaded convenience item requiring microwave cooking or heating), 1/2–1 cup starch (potato, rice, or pasta), and 1/2 cup green or yellow vegetable; diet iced tea
- Physical activity: Moderate amounts of walking, lifting, and stacking greeting cards and display racks for five to six hours

Non-workdays

- Wakes at 8:30 AM
- Breakfast: Same as workdays
- Lunch: Same as workdays
- Evening meal: Same as workdays, but meat/poultry/fish is usually baked or roasted, fewer convenience items. Has added dinner roll and occasional dessert—few (three or four) regular cookies or 1/2 cup ice cream
- Eats pizza every Friday: Two slices (pepperoni or mushroom) with tossed salad, 2 tablespoons regular dressing, diet soda, and no dessert
- Physical activity: not as strenuous as workdays, mostly chores such as grocery shopping, errands, laundry, house cleaning (shared with husband; Barbara does light duties, husband does vacuuming)

Situation

Barbara knows the basics of carbohydrate counting and tries to follow guidelines for specific servings at each meal. She admits to not always paying attention to portions and sometimes eating more or less than her allotted servings. Barbara has had a 10-pound weight gain in the past five years. She checks her blood glucose four times a day and has erratic results. Her fasting levels are usually within her target range, but her preprandial glucose levels range from the 70–350 mg/dl. Her A1C values in the past year have been slightly higher than she prefers: 7.9%, 7.8%, and 7.8%. She complains of more frequent hypoglycemia in the afternoons on the days she is more active at work, usually two days a week. She realizes she overtreats her hypoglycemia while working because she is too busy to stop and recheck her blood sugar and is concerned about becoming unconscious at work. Barbara stated, "I just keep eating until I feel better, and then by the time I get home, I'm high and I have to take more insulin before dinner. That insulin makes me feel hungry, so I end up eating a lot more than I planned to on those days."

Barbara wants to improve her A1C values, prevent the "blood sugar swings," lose weight, and prevent or reduce her hypoglycemic episodes. She and her physician have decided that pump therapy, or continuous subcutaneous insulin infusion (CSII), would provide Barbara the flexibility she needs and offer her more options for managing her diabetes and meal choices. Barbara's physician and she discussed her fasting and preprandial target blood glucose levels and developed the following:

- Fasting level of 100 mg/dl
- Two- to three-hour postprandial of <180 mg/dl, ideally <160 mg/dl

Barbara's physician referred her to the dietitian at the local diabetes center to learn Advanced Carbohydrate Counting in preparation for CSII therapy. Barbara would like to begin CSII sometime in the next five months, before a scheduled 10-day cruise to celebrate her 25th wedding anniversary. After learning Advanced Carbohydrate Counting, Barbara will contact several pump company manufacturers to obtain information. She will also meet with a certified diabetes educator (CDE) at the diabetes center to learn more about CSII.

Barbara made an appointment to meet with the dietitian. She agreed to keep one week of records of SMBG results, insulin doses, food intake, hypoglycemic treatment, and physical activity.

Dietitian's Action Plan

1. Discuss carbohydrate count of Barbara's meals, including dinner convenience items and actual amounts versus Barbara's recollections of 1/2 cup portions of rice and pasta. Remind Barbara to pay attention to the Nutrition Facts panel on food labels to figure out the amount of carbohydrate in her portions as compared with the label serving sizes. Ask Barbara to measure foods to confirm her portions (such as juice, cereals, rice, and pasta).

2. Download Barbara's meter. Review her results and correlate with her food records. Point out the differences in the carbohydrate amounts and relate effects to specific insulin doses.

3. Explain the concepts of matching insulin to carbohydrate amounts and correcting elevated blood glucose levels with a specific amount of insulin that lowers a specific amount of glucose.

4. Develop ICR and CF based on her records. Use an average of her rapid-acting insulin preprandial doses and supplemental doses and add to her bedtime glargine dose to derive her TDD.

   Breakfast: 9 units

   Lunch: 10 units

   Evening meal: 13 units

   Bedtime: 26 units

   TDD: 59 units

   Calculate her ICR using food records and insulin doses. For example, her breakfast carbohydrate totals and usual insulin dose:

   8 ounces orange juice = 30 grams of carbohydrate

   One bowl corn flakes or granola cereal = 30 grams of carbohydrate

   8 ounces 2% milk = 12 grams of carbohydrate

   Coffee with sugar substitute = 0 grams of carbohydrate

   Total carbohydrate grams = 72 grams

   Average insulin dose = 9 units

   72 grams of carbohydrate ÷ 9 units of insulin = 8 grams/unit

   Using food records and insulin doses, determine that Barbara's ICR is one unit to 8 grams of carbohydrate, or 1:8. Compare with using the Rule of 500:

   500 ÷ TDD (57) = 8.9, round to 9

   ICR is 1:9

   Since Barbara's postprandial glucose and A1C values are elevated, the dietitian suggested using 1:8 as Barbara's ICR, since this would provide slightly more insulin coverage for the total amount of carbohydrate in Barbara's meals.

   To determine the CF, they used the 1800 Rule, dividing 1800 by her TDD:

   1800 ÷ 57 = 31.5, round to 30

   CF is 30 mg/dl

5. Discuss when and how to use her ICR and CF formulas, including how to adapt the formulas to differing carbohydrate content. Ask Barbara to practice using her formulas to calculate sample meal doses and correction doses of insulin.

Since Barbara has steadily gained weight over the past few years, suggest healthier food choices to assist with weight loss, such as 1% or skim milk instead of 2% milk at breakfast; reduced-calorie dressing or less regular dressing; and more non-breaded convenience dinner entrees.

6. Ask Barbara to mail or fax one week of records, including carbohydrate gram amounts, portions, insulin doses, SMBG values, and any changes in activity levels. Also include foods (carbohydrate grams and type of food/beverage) used to treat her hypoglycemia. Schedule a call to review the records Barbara provided.

Barbara's Goals

Based on the meeting with the dietitian, Barbara set the following goals.

1. Begin using her ICR and CF to calculate preprandial insulin doses.

2. Keep detailed records, as discussed with the dietitian.

3. Try to incorporate the healthier food choices suggested by the dietitian.

4. Measure actual portions of juices, cereals, rice, and pasta at home using measuring equipment in her kitchen.

Follow-Up

1. Barbara's mailed records indicated occasional postprandial glucose levels of 180–200 mg/dl, but most blood glucose values improved, often falling within 30 mg/dl of her preprandial target of 100 mg/dl. She also reported fewer episodes of hypoglycemia and the "big swings" that had resulted from overtreatment.

2. After measuring some of her favorite foods, Barbara realized she was consuming larger portions of rice and pasta than she previously thought. Her estimated 1/2-cup portions were actually 1 cup portions.

3. Closely reading food labels helped Barbara realize that her granola cereal portion, though similar in size to her corn flakes portion, contained much more carbohydrate than corn flakes. She began to look at other cereals in the grocery store to compare carbohydrate values. Since she was concerned with weight, she decided to choose cereals with a lower carbohydrate content than granola.

4. After six weeks of using her ICR and CF, Barbara called the dietitian to meet again for additional review of some "trouble spots" (e.g., blood glu-

cose values after pizza and on days with higher activity). An appointment was set for two weeks later. Barbara also made an appointment the same week with another CDE at the diabetes center to look at the various insulin pump models. Barbara felt confident that she would be ready to begin the process of choosing a pump and initiating the insurance paperwork and coverage. If things went as planned, Barbara would be using pump therapy two months before her anniversary cruise!

CASE STUDY #3: BILL

History
Bill is a 35-year-old married graphic arts designer who has had type 1 diabetes for 24 years. He has worn an insulin pump for eight years. Bill has had "pretty good" control with CSII, but has noticed his glucose levels have been a bit more erratic the past two years. His A1C values have increased from the high 6% range to the mid 7% range (7.5% and 7.7%) in the past six months.

Data
Ht: 5'10"; Wt: 175 pounds; Weight increase of 6 pounds in the past year, previous weight stable.

Food Habits and Daily Schedule
Workdays:
  Wakes at 6:30 AM
  • Breakfast: 7:15–7:30 AM: Stops at fast food restaurant three days a week; has fried egg with slice of Canadian bacon on English muffin and coffee with half-and-half and sugar substitute; other two days has small bowl of oat bran cereal with about 1/2 cup of 1% milk and coffee.
  • Lunch: 11:30–12 Noon: Occasionally brings sandwich from home prepared by his wife: two slices white or wheat bread with two slices leftover meat or chicken, mayonnaise, and lettuce; diet soda. Several days a week, eats in local diner or restaurant—"basic meat, starch, vegetable meal with diet iced tea."
  • Evening meal: 7:00 PM: Prepared by Bill's wife: tossed salad with 1–2 tablespoons diet salad dressing, meat, poultry, or fish, grilled or roasted, 1 cup starch, such as potatoes, pasta, or rice, 1/2 cup green vegetable, juice-packed or fresh fruit for dessert, diet soda or iced tea
  • Bedtime snack, between 9:30 and 10:30 PM: fresh fruit, pretzels, or 2–3 cookies; occasional 1/2 cup ice cream or sherbet

- Physical activity: Light amount of walking each evening when he walks the family dog after dinner

Weekend/non-workdays:
- Wakes at 8:30 AM
- Breakfast: 8:30 to 9:00 AM: Small bowl of oat bran cereal with about 1/2 cup of 1% milk and coffee or 2–3 times/month has larger breakfast at restaurant, usually French toast with syrup or scrambled eggs with bacon and toast, coffee
- Lunch: Variable, sometimes skips lunch when running errands; if has lunch, eats sub-style sandwich with assorted deli meats and cheeses and diet soda.
- Evening meal: 7:00 PM: Prepared by Bill's wife: Similar to weekday meals: tossed salad with 1–2 tablespoons diet salad dressing, meat, poultry, or fish, grilled or roasted, 1 cup starch, such as potatoes, pasta, or rice, 1/2 cup green vegetable, juice-packed or fresh fruit for dessert, diet soda or iced tea. Occasionally (1 to 2 times/month) has restaurant meal, often Chinese or Mexican. Has "more carbs than usual."
- Bedtime snack, between 9:30 and 10:30 PM: Fresh fruit, pretzels, or 2–3 cookies; occasional 1/2 cup ice cream or sherbet
- Physical activity: Plays golf two Saturdays/month; light amount of walking each evening when he walks the family dog after dinner

Regimen
Insulin aspart via CSII. Recent 30-day average of TDD has been 41 units/day. Basal rates total 20.7 units/day.
  Profile in units:
  12 AM–3 AM: 0.8
  3 AM–7 AM: 1.1
  7 AM–10 AM: 0.9
  10 AM–12 AM: 0.8
  ICR is 1:12 and CF is 50 mg/dl.
  Boluses are 18 to 25 units/day (average of 21 units/day).

Situation
Bill noticed his fasting blood glucose readings are usually 30+ mg/dl within his target of 100 mg/dl, but his pre-lunch, pre-dinner, and bedtime readings have become elevated. Because of this, he has been using more correction boluses than usual. Bill is also eating more than he had in the past and thinks this is due to both a change in his job duties, where he sits at a desk more often and snacks more often, as well as eating to "chase" the insulin if he overcorrects. At his last

appointment four months earlier, Bill's endocrinologist increased Bill's daytime basal rate to 0.8 units/hour (from 0.7 units/hour). At his physician's request, Bill conducted several basal check tests (fasted for four to six hours in different blocks of time throughout the day over several days and checked blood glucose hourly) to confirm his basal rate was appropriate. During the basal check tests, Bill's glucose levels stayed within 30 mg/dl from the beginning and throughout the basal checking period, which confirmed his basal rate was keeping his glucose in a steady range. Bill meets quarterly with his endocrinologist for his routine appointment. At his last appointment, the endocrinologist referred him to a local dietitian, CDE for a review of carbohydrate counting; both Bill and his physician believe that Bill may need a higher ICR.

Dietitian's Action Plan

1. Bill scheduled an appointment to meet with the dietitian. She asked that he bring a week's worth of records of his SMBG results, meals and snacks with portions sizes and calculated carbohydrate grams, meal boluses, correction boluses, hypoglycemic episodes and treatments, activity notes, and any other pertinent information to help analyze his management.

2. Bill and the dietitian met. She reviewed his records and determined Bill was accurate in his carbohydrate counting technique, but noted he used two to three daily correction boluses. She suggested he increase his ICR from 1:12 to 1:10. By doing this, Bill's meal boluses would be increased.

3. Bill agreed to try using a 1:10 ICR for a few days to see if this made a difference with his preprandial lunch and dinner and bedtime glucose levels. He agreed to keep a few days of records and fax his results to the dietitian.

Follow-Up

1. Bill faxed five days of records to the dietitian. Upon review, she noted that Bill had several one-hour postprandial glucose levels that were in the 70s and 60s (mg/dl) followed by two- and three-hour postprandial readings in the low to mid 200s (mg/dl). When Bill experienced hypoglycemia, he treated it appropriately, but then had much higher readings at the next meal.

2. When the dietitian spoke with Bill, he verbalized his frustration. "When I take a little more insulin to cover my carbs, I go too low and I end up eating more to treat that, and then I end up higher before the next meal.

I don't think this is working too well. My old ratio of 1:12 wasn't working too well either. I'm just frustrated with the crazy numbers."

3. The dietitian told Bill about a medication, pramlintide, that could help him with his high postprandial blood glucose levels. She explained that pramlintide is injected before meals and worked to lower postprandial glucose levels by suppressing postprandial glucagon secretion and by slowing the time it took food to leave the stomach—essentially slowing down the rate at which it hits his bloodstream as glucose. She said pramlintide could lower his blood glucose levels after meals and also help him feel full so that he might not feel as hungry, which could help him cut down on the between-meal snacking. She suggested Bill call his endocrinologist to discuss adding pramlintide to his regimen at his next visit. She also gave Bill the website information for pramlintide so he could look into this on his own before meeting with his endocrinologist.

Bill was interested in trying pramlintide. He realized he wasn't looking forward to injections, as he really enjoyed CSII over multiple daily injection (MDI) therapy, but he was willing to try pramlintide. Bill understood if pramlintide could make a difference in "smoothing out" his blood glucose numbers and decreasing his appetite, taking a small injection before each of his meals wouldn't be an issue.

Bill's Goals

Based on the follow-up with the dietitian, Bill set the following goals.

1. Call his physician for an appointment to discuss the use of pramlintide.
2. Review information about Symlin via the website provided by the dietitian.
3. Return to using his previous ratio of 1:12.

Action Plan

1. Bill met with his physician to discuss adding pramlintide to his regimen. The endocrinologist agreed that adding pramlintide might be helpful. He also explained that pramlintide may cause nausea the first few days, but the nausea is usually mild and lessens over time. Bill was told that he would need to cut back his meal boluses by 50% to reduce potential insulin-induced hypoglycemia. The endocrinologist advised Bill that pramlintide alone does not cause low blood glucose, but when added to insulin, the normal insulin dose could cause low blood glucose. Reducing his prandial boluses meant Bill would need less insulin to cover carbohydrate. Because of this, he would use an ICR of 1:24 instead of 1:12.

2. Bill was provided with a starter kit for pramlintide and a prescription for pramlintide. He was advised to schedule an appointment with the dietitian for the initiation of his pramlintide, adjustment of his ICR, and a refresher on injection therapy.

3. Bill met with the dietitian, CDE. She explained how pramlintide worked and advised Bill that he may actually experience hyperglycemia the first few days after starting pramlintide due to cutting back on his mealtime insulin, but this was just temporary. She then reviewed the pramlintide titration schedule with Bill:

    - Start with a dose of 15 mcg; increase the dose by 15 mcg every three to seven days (or when the nausea, if present, disappears) to reach the maintenance dose, which is 60 mcg for a person with type 1 diabetes.
    - Pramlintide should be injected at the start of a meal that contains at least 30 grams of carbohydrate or 250 calories.
    - Reduce mealtime insulin by 50%; for Bill, that means using an ICR of 1: 24 instead of 1:12.
    - Call or fax the dietitian every three to four days with blood glucose results. She will advise Bill about gradually increasing his ICR from 1:24 to maybe 1:20, or even 1:18, depending on his glucose results.
    - Follow the titration schedule for the next few weeks and adjust the pramlintide and insulin gradually per the dietitian's instructions until the blood glucose levels are within Bill's target range.

Bill verbalized understanding of the dosing and was eager to start using Symlin.

Follow-Up

After five weeks of using pramlintide, Bill contacted the dietitian, CDE for a follow-up.

1. Bill had a bit of nausea the first two days using pramlintide. He described the nausea as "feeling full, like after eating a Thanksgiving dinner, not feeling like I was going to throw up." He kept in close contact with either the dietitian or another CDE at the diabetes center. The dietitian advised Bill when to increase his pramlintide dose and gradually increase his ICR.

2. Bill followed the pramlintide titration schedule and is taking 60 mcg pramlintide before each breakfast, lunch, and evening meal.

3. The dietitian gradually increased Bill's ICR two days after titrating up his pramlintide dose. After three weeks, Bill's new ICR is 1:18.

4. Bill is very pleased with his blood glucose results. He has fewer fluctuations and less hypoglycemia, as well as less hyperglycemia.

Follow-Up

After three months using pramlintide in conjunction with his CSII, Bill reported back.

1. His pramlintide therapy seemed to be going well and he described his current situation:
   - A1C: 7.1%, decreased 0.6 % from 7.7%
   - Weight: 171 pounds, decreased 4 pounds from 175 pounds
   - ICR: 1 unit to 18 grams of carbohydrate, decreased from 1:12 and 1:10
   - CF: same (50 mg/dl), but used less frequently
   - Basal rates: same (20.7 units/day)
   - Bolus doses: average of 15 units/day, a decrease of about 25% overall from average of 21 units/day

2. Bill told both his endocrinologist and the dietitian he is very happy with the improvements in his diabetes. He is eating less and feels much better about his control, due to fewer fluctuations in his blood glucose numbers. Bill is also pleased that he has better control, a lower A1C and has also lost weight in about three months' time.

Related Topics

CHAPTER TEN

Impact on Glycemia of Dietary Components Beyond Carbohydrate

It is recognized that dietary carbohydrate is the major determinant of postprandial glucose levels (ADA 2008b). However, it is also known that other dietary components and myriad interrelated factors, several of which are noted in Table I-2 on page 3 in the introduction, further influence postprandial and overall blood glucose control. In addition to the factors listed in this table, one can add the effect of the volume of food intake, pace of eating, and timing of bolus insulin to cover food intake. A small amount of research and expert consensus provide guidance in these areas, however, much remains to be researched and learned.

This chapter will focus on many of the predominant determinants of postprandial and overall blood glucose control other than carbohydrate, including protein and fat, the glycemic index, dietary fiber, the effects of body weight, restaurant meals, sugar alcohols, and alcohol.

SOURCES OF PROTEIN AND FAT

For some time there was a common notion that 50% of ingested protein was converted into glucose, but this has been disputed by research (ADA 2008b; Franz 2000). Current research and consensus indicates that, in people with type 1 diabetes, protein has little effect on blood glucose response when consumed in commonly eaten amounts (3–4 ounces), though very large portions may affect glucose (ADA 2008b). Larger than usual amounts of protein have been shown to cause both a slower and greater than expected rise in blood glucose level (Gannon et al. 2001). In individuals with type 2 diabetes, ingested protein does not increase plasma glucose response, but does increase serum insulin responses (ADA 2008b; Franz 2000). However, it is also speculated that the insulin response stimulated by the dietary protein consumed causes the glucose formed to be rapidly stored as glycogen in the liver and skeletal muscles (ADA 2008b).

The impact of fat on postprandial blood glucose is generally to delay the rise of glucose, but not to cause a greater than expected rise (Franz 2000; Gannon et al. 2001). This may be because fat delays gastric emptying, which in turn slows glucose absorption (Peters and Davidson 1993; Jones et al. 2005). Other factors also may play a role, such as a slower gastric emptying if blood glucose is high, the size of the meal, with larger meals taking longer to raise blood glucose, the pace with which a meal is eaten, and other dietary factors (Jones et al. 2005).

At this point there are no published guidelines for what to teach people with diabetes about managing high protein and/or fat meals. However, there is general agreement about the following educational points:

- Educate people that if they eat a desirable amount of protein-based foods (meats) at a meal (2–4 ounces cooked) with moderate amounts of other sources of protein, this is likely to have minimal impact on postprandial blood glucose.
- When a person eats a larger-than-usual portion of meat, and in particular, high-fat sources of meat (as a result of either cut or preparation), they should anticipate that their blood glucose will rise more slowly and possibly to a higher degree (due to the high protein content). Whereas a more desirable amount of meat within a common meal would cause a peak rise in blood glucose 1–2 hours after a meal, a meal with a large amount of protein and fat may cause a peak a number of hours after that.
- For healthy eating and glycemic control, protein content at meals should be based on personal caloric needs.

People need to know that the impact of meals with high amounts of protein and fat on postprandial blood glucose will vary from person to person and situation to situation. Encourage people to learn their individual responses to meals they commonly eat and use a variety of techniques to manage these situations. Some people may find they need more insulin to cover a meal with both high protein and fat, but not a high-protein, low-fat meal.

Fat and protein impact on insulin therapy

For those using continuous subcutaneous insulin infusion (CSII), two meal studies have demonstrated that using a combination bolus was the most effective way to manage postprandial glucose. One study in people using CSII and eating pizza, showed that using a 50/50 combination bolus (50% immediate bolus, 50% extended bolus) over eight hours most effectively controlled postprandial glucose

(Jones et al. 2005). Another study using a moderate-carbohydrate, low-protein, and moderate-to-high-fat meal, showed that using a 70% immediate bolus and a 30% extended-over-90-minute bolus, most effectively managed postprandial glucose (Chase et al. 2002).

People need to be provided with techniques to manage various situations (Warshaw 2005). The techniques they put to use will also be dependent on how they deliver insulin. People using multiple daily injection (MDI) therapy might try mimicking an insulin pump combination dose, splitting their bolus dose and taking some insulin prior to the meal and some about an hour or so after the start of the meal. Chapter 7 provides more detail on dosing options.

GLYCEMIC INDEX AND LOAD

Glycemic index and glycemic load are two concepts that have been developed over the last few decades to compare the postprandial responses to constant amounts of different carbohydrate-containing foods (ADA 2008b; Sheard et al. 2004). The glycemic index of a food is defined as the increase over fasting blood glucose it elicits two hours after ingestion of a constant amount of that food (usually a 50-gram carbohydrate portion) divided by the response to a reference food (usually glucose or white bread). The glycemic load of foods, meals, and diets are calculated by multiplying the glycemic index of the constituent foods by the amounts of carbohydrate in each food and then totaling the values for all foods (ADA 2008b).

Over the years there has been much published and debated about the use of these concepts in diabetes meal planning. Several randomized clinical trials have reported that low glycemic index diets reduce glycemia in diabetic subjects (Brand-Miller et al. 2003), but, according to several review papers, other clinical trials have not confirmed this effect (ADA 2008b; Sheard et al. 2004). The American Diabetes Association (ADA) Nutrition Recommendations state, "Thus, it appears that low glycemic index diets can produce a modest benefit in controlling postprandial hyperglycemia." The recommendations do reiterate that total carbohydrate remains the major factor to impact postprandial blood glucose (ADA 2008b). Educators may want to teach people that the glycemic index or load of a food is one more factor to consider when choosing foods, however, evidence suggests that the focus of carbohydrate-counting education should be on total carbohydrate.

Educators should keep several other points in mind as they discuss these concepts. The glycemic index of foods is available only for commonly eaten, non-mixed foods; once foods or ingredients become mixed, glycemic index numbers are less applicable. In other words, oats, beans, pasta, carrots, watermelon, and potatoes have been assigned a glycemic index number on several glycemic index charts, but casseroles and mixed dishes have not. Several charts are available and there is variability in the glycemic index of foods between these charts. As of this publishing, one list can be accessed at *www.diabetesnet.com/diabetes_food_diet/ glycemic_index.php*.

It's also important to note that the type of carbohydrate (e.g., starch or sugar) does not consistently predict the glycemic index. For example, some fruits have a low glycemic index (apples and oranges) and others have a higher glycemic index (watermelon and pineapple). The glycemic index also does not provide an indication of the nutrient composition or quality of the food. For this reason, people should not necessarily be discouraged from eating foods that provide a quality nutrient source simply because they have a high glycemic index or glycemic load, especially if this limits the breadth of nutritious foods people enjoy. People should also be taught that food-related factors other than glycemic index can affect blood glucose levels, adding to the complexity of blood glucose control.

Lastly, because there can be so much variability in individual foods and people's response to them, encourage people to develop their own "personal glycemic index." Suggest that as they progress with carbohydrate counting and learn more

Table 10-1. Factors That Affect Postprandial Blood Glucose

- Ripeness of the food (the riper the food, the more quickly it can raise blood glucose)

- Form the food is eaten in—raw or cooked—and if it is cooked, how well it is cooked (the more a food is cooked, the more likely it is to raise blood glucose quickly)

- Variety of the food (for example, long grain or short grain rice, Yukon Gold or red potato, when and where a product was grown)

- Amount of fiber, fructose, lactose, and fat in the meal (these tend to slow glycemic response) (ADA 2008b)

- Individual responses to foods and different responses on different days

- Other foods eaten at the meal or snack

- Blood glucose at the time of eating

- Sequencing of food-related medication and food

- Level of insulin resistance (overall and time of day)

about the impact of various foods and meals on their blood glucose and that they use these results to make adjustments in their medication.

ADJUSTING FOR DIETARY FIBER INTAKE

People with diabetes are encouraged, like all individuals, to increase their intake of fiber to reach a goal of 14 grams per 1000 kcal, or about 21–38 grams per day for various adult age groups (Institute of Medicine 2002). To achieve this goal people should choose a variety of fiber-containing foods, such as legumes, fiber-rich cereals (>5 grams of fiber per serving), fruits, vegetables, and whole-grain products that also provide vitamins, minerals, and other substances (ADA 2008b); U.S. Department of Health and Human Services 2005). In terms of the impact of fiber on glycemia and lipids, the data suggest that people would need to consume much larger amounts (~50 grams fiber per day) than the current average of about 10–14 grams/day to achieve these goals (ADA 2008b). It is important to help people realize that, on average, Americans only eat about half the amount of dietary fiber they need.

Subtracting fiber from carbohydrate counts

There has been much debate about whether people who learn carbohydrate counting should be taught to subtract the amount of fiber from a food or meal from the total carbohydrate count to determine their medication dose (generally their bolus rapid-acting insulin). The rationale for teaching this concept is that the grams of dietary fiber from the total carbohydrate count are, for the most part, not digested and absorbed as glucose. However, the majority of people learning carbohydrate counting, especially those with type 2 diabetes using Basic Carbohydrate Counting, cannot apply and/or don't need to be taught this concept.

Rather than spending time teaching this concept to all people who learn carbohydrate counting, it is more logical to teach this concept only to people who fit one or more of these four categories:

1. Eats a high-fiber diet (>14 grams/1000 kcal) and/or regularly eats specifically high-fiber foods that are individually or cumulatively more than 5 grams of fiber per food (e.g., high-fiber cereal) or per meal (e.g., brown rice, beans with whole-grain tortillas)

2. Demonstrates excellent accuracy in carbohydrate-counting skills

3. Is able to easily and quickly do the math involved in these calculations

4. Uses a blood glucose–lowering medication that can be adjusted for the fiber content and may put them at risk of hypoglycemia

Subtracting Fiber

The following is an example of how to factor in the dietary fiber content of a meal that contains several sources of dietary fiber. Note that this guideline is in sync with the recommendation in *Choose Your Foods: Exchange Lists for Diabetes* (ADA, American Dietetic Association, 2007), which states: "If a food contains more than 5 grams of fiber, subtract half the grams of fiber from the carbohydrate grams to get the total carbohydrate grams." This same logic can be applied to meals with a fiber content greater than 5 grams in total.

A high-fiber breakfast:	Carbohydrate(g)	Fiber (g)
1 cup high-fiber flake cereal	32	6
One slice whole grain bread	12	3
1 cup nonfat milk	12	2
1 1/4 cup strawberries	15	2
Total	**71**	**11**

½ grams of dietary fiber = 6

Subtract 6 grams of fiber from the 71 grams of carbohydrate. Figure the insulin dose of rapid-acting insulin based on 65 g of carbohydrate (71 − 6 = 65 grams).

See the box Subtracting Fiber for an example of how subtracting the fiber content from total carbohydrate could be done.

TREATING HYPOGLYCEMIA

As educators work with people with diabetes who take blood glucose–lowering medications, it is important to determine a person's risk for hypoglycemia, which ADA defines as under 70 mg/dl (plasma glucose) (ADA 2008a). Today some blood glucose–lowering medications do and others do not cause hypoglycemia. (Chapter 12 provides a review of blood glucose–lowering medications.) Hypoglycemia can occur in people treated with insulin therapy and/or an insulin secretagogue (including sulfonylureas, meglintinides, and D-phenylalanines). Also, because people with diabetes often have unwarranted fears about hypoglycemia and therefore resist intensive glycemic control, it is important to stress the relative likelihood and frequency of hypoglycemia and put undue fears to rest (Polonsky and Jackson 2004).

Most episodes of hypoglycemia can be effectively self-treated provided the person is of the age and ability to treat themselves. People should be encouraged to use the 15/15 guideline initially. However, if a person is using Advanced Carbohydrate Counting and their insulin-to-carbohydrate ratio (ICR) varies more than a few grams of carbohydrate from 15, encourage them to use their ICR to treat hypoglycemia instead (e.g., if their ICR is 1:20, then they may need 20 grams of carbohydrate to raise their blood glucose enough).

Teach people to consume about 15 grams of glucose to treat hypoglycemia. It's preferable to use a source of glucose, such as glucose tablets or gels that are 100% glucose, as opposed to other carbohydrates (ADA 2008b). Glycemic response correlates better with the glucose, however, any form of carbohydrate that contains glucose may be used.

Treatment should take effect in 15 minutes. However, this may only temporarily raise blood glucose. For this reason, teach people to recheck their blood glucose in 15 minutes to determine the need to repeat the treatment. Blood glucose is likely to rise faster when hypoglycemic because gastric emptying and absorption is more rapid (Chase et al. 2002; Jones et al. 2005).

ADA points out that adding a source of protein to the glucose source doesn't affect the glycemic response or prevent subsequent hypoglycemia (ADA 2008b). Educators should not continue to teach this concept because it is not supported by research. In people with type 2 diabetes, ingested protein does not increase plasma glucose response, but does increase serum insulin responses and thus shouldn't be used to treat acute hypoglycemia or prevent nighttime hypoglycemia (ADA 2008b). Also, remind people not to use chocolate candy or other food with a high fat content to treat hypoglycemia, because the fat component can delay the rise of blood glucose.

WEIGHT MANAGEMENT

As people improve glycemic control, there has been a documented potential for unwanted weight gain. People in the intensive group of the Diabetes Control and Complications Trial (DCCT) gained an average of 10 pounds during the first year of the trial (DCCT Research Group 1993; DCCT Research Group 1997). Weight gain that accompanies improved glycemic control can be attributed to several factors:

- The loss of fewer calories from glycosuria
- Normalizing of glycemia promotes rehydration
- Greater frequency of hypoglycemia and need to treat it
- Underestimates of carbohydrate content consumed
- Use of one or more glucose-lowering medications that are known to cause weight gain

There is conjecture that people who use carbohydrate counting as their meal planning method may have been either uninformed or not cognizant of the calories from protein and fat and/or might experiment with the inclusion of higher-calorie foods. One or both situations will increase calorie intake and result in weight gain. It is ideal to let people who are striving to achieve glycemic control know that weight gain is a possibility.

To prevent undesired weight gain provide people with guidelines for the consumption of protein and fat (see guidelines on Table 3-1, pages 22–23). Encourage people to be aware of the protein and fat content of their meals and to recognize that while they can take more insulin or medication to "cover" the glycemic rise from sweets, these foods still have calories and overconsumption can result in weight gain.

RESTAURANT FOODS AND MEALS

Today people eat, on average, five meals a week away from home (National Restaurant Association 2008), and are spending approximately half their food dollar away from home. For many people these numbers are even higher and trend data predicts continued growth in dollars spent away from home. When educators ask people about their consumption of restaurant meals, they should consider meals eaten in restaurants as well as those taken out or ordered from restaurants. Eating restaurant foods both inside and outside of restaurants has become commonplace, both as a means of consuming quick and convenient meals and socializing. The potential for larger than desirable portions, higher intake of sugars and fats, and lower intake of fruit, vegetables, and whole grains in restaurant meals has been documented in numerous publications (Pereira et al. 2005; Bowman and Vinyard 2004). Clearly, these factors can affect a person's health and make healthy restaurant eating a challenge.

In an effort to personalize education on healthy eating and restaurant foods, educators should ascertain:

- how often the person eats restaurant foods/meals,
- the types of restaurant foods/meals the person eats,
- food choices at/from the various restaurants,
- and willingness and ability to change current habits.

With this information the educator can prioritize how important knowledge about restaurant eating is and individualize teaching based on the types of restaurants frequented and the food choices made. If the educator is teaching in a group setting, the educator can gather information in the same manner and teach based on general needs of the audience. The more often someone eats out, the more important it will be to develop guidelines for healthy eating and estimating carbohydrate counts in restaurants.

General strategies for healthy restaurant eating can also be provided. People need to know how to limit the amount of carbohydrate, protein, and fat they consume, and how to practice portion control (see tips for controlling restaurant portions on page 36 in chapter 4). For example, if a person eats three lunches a week at a fast food hamburger chain and their usual order is a double cheeseburger, large fries, and diet beverage, the educator can:

1. help the person realize the amount of calories and grams of carbohydrate they consume in this or other restaurant meals (oftentimes raising awareness is the best teacher);

2. help the person think about how they can reduce the number of fast food meals they consume;

3. discuss healthier food choices at the restaurant using nutrition information from that restaurant if it is available;

4. suggest alternative restaurants that serve a wider variety of healthier options;

5. and/or provide carbohydrate information for that restaurant chain or information about how to access it.

Perhaps the most important skill is learning about resources and using these to obtain the carbohydrate counts of the foods. This information can also help in estimating the carbohydrate counts of the foods for which there is no information. People who eat certain ethnic fare, such as Asian cuisines, need to know that dishes may contain sugar, cornstarch, or sauces that contain carbohydrate. Encourage people to weigh and measure foods at home and to use the Hand Guides for Portion Control on page 34 in chapter 4 to closely estimate portions and therefore carbohydrate counts.

Resources to obtain the carbohydrate counts of restaurant foods and consumer resources to help with strategies for restaurant eating are listed in Appendix I. People can easily gain access to the carbohydrate counts and other nutrition information for foods served by many of the large national chain restaurants. This includes restaurants serving hamburgers, chicken, pizza, Mexican food, coffee shops, salad/sandwich shops, and bagel bakeries. Information is available online (see Appendix I for hints about accessing), on the walls of restaurants, or in brochures or pocket guides. Much less information is available from sit-down style national chain restaurants and independent restaurants.

People should be encouraged to check their blood glucose level more often when they eat restaurant foods. These additional SMBG checks can provide valuable information, including

- the effect extra food has on the amount and timing of postprandial glucose levels;
- how nutrient composition and pace at which the meal is eaten affects glucose levels;
- and data on the effect of certain types of food on blood glucose levels, i.e., Chinese, Mexican, pizza, etc.

FOODS THAT CONTAIN POLYOLS (SUGAR ALCOHOLS)

Polyols, frequently referred to as sugar alcohols (though they are not sucrose or alcohol-based), are a group of ingredients commonly used in some "sugar-free" foods. Polyols are used to replace sucrose-containing ingredients in foods such as candy, cookies, and ice creams. Today, these ingredients may be used alone in foods or combined with sucrose-containing ingredients or no-calorie sweeteners. Common names are isomalt, sorbitol, lactitol, maltitol, mannitol, and xylitol. A common two-letter ending for these ingredients is "ol." This is a good guideline to provide to those searching for these ingredients on an ingredients label.

Polyols contain about half the calories of sucrose-containing ingredients (4 kcal/g) and produce a lower postprandial glucose response than sucrose or glucose. The intake of polyols by the general public and people with diabetes is safe. However, the ADA suggests that there is no evidence that correlates the amount of polyols likely to be consumed with a reduction in glycemia, energy intake, or weight (ADA 2008b), mostly because people don't use these foods frequently enough to result in a significant impact and the calories and grams of carbohydrate per serving of sugar-free foods sweetened with polyols are often only minimally reduced.

A downside of polyols is that in large amounts and in some people they can cause gas, cramps, and/or diarrhea. Some people, especially children, may be bothered by this side effect. Foods with certain amounts of polyols must contain information on the label about this possible "laxative effect" (ADA 2008b; Warshaw and Powers 1999).

ADA suggests that when people use foods that contain polyols, that they subtract half the grams of polyols (sugar alcohols) from the total carbohydrate listed on the Nutrition Facts panel (ADA 2008b). Educators can also choose to use the following guidelines (Warshaw and Powers 1999):

- If the food contains several sources of carbohydrate, including polyols, subtract half of the grams of polyols from the total carbohydrate grams. Figure the remaining grams of carbohydrate into the eating plan.

- If all the carbohydrate in the food is from polyols and the grams of polyols are >10, subtract half of the grams of polyols from the total carbohydrate grams. Figure the remaining carbohydrate grams into the eating plan.

- If all the carbohydrate in the food is from polyols and/or no-calorie sweeteners and the total carbohydrates are <10 grams, consider it a free food.

Perhaps the most important message for educators to teach is to compare the Nutrition Facts panel with the similar sucrose-containing food. Oftentimes the calorie and carbohydrate savings is marginal.

ALCOHOL

People with diabetes can choose to drink alcohol. From a health standpoint the same guidelines that apply to the general population apply to people with diabetes (U.S. Department of Health and Human Services 2005). Alcohol intake should be moderate and is defined as one drink per day or less for women and two drinks per day or less for men. A drink is defined as 12 ounces of beer, 5 ounces of wine, or 1.5 ounces distilled spirits. Each contains about 15 grams of alcohol (ADA 2008b). Some people should not consume alcohol, including people with a history of alcohol abuse, medical problems such as severe hypertriglyceridemia, or women who are pregnant (ADA 2008b).

Alcohol does not require insulin for metabolism. Pure alcohol, such as whiskey, gin, rum, or vodka contains calories but not carbohydrate. Moderate amounts of alcohol, when ingested with food, have minimal impact on plasma glucose. However, alcohol can cause a rise in blood glucose if an excess of alcohol is consumed, and any carbohydrate that is consumed with the alcohol, either in the alcoholic drink or as food, can raise blood glucose. People who take any form of insulin or a blood glucose–lowering medication that can cause hypoglycemia (see Appendix II) should be made aware that alcohol can also cause hypoglycemia.

To prevent hypoglycemia, people should be encouraged to ingest a form of carbohydrate when they consume alcohol. People should also be educated that if they consume alcohol during the evening, the most common time for alcohol intake, they are more at risk for hypoglycemia during the night or even as late as the next morning. Alcohol can have a delayed blood glucose–lowering effect as much as 12 hours later (ADA 2008b).

Educate people to think about when and what they are drinking. Advise people to review beer, wine, and wine spritzer labels and to learn the amount of carbohydrate in alcoholic beverages. Some may find that light beer, dry wine, and drinks made with non-caloric mixers may require little or no medication/insulin adjustments. Teach people whether they can or cannot be at risk for hypoglycemia based on the blood glucose–lowering medication they take. Encourage them to be aware of their blood glucose level as well as the status of their blood glucose–lowering medication at the time of alcohol consumption. Also encourage vigilance with checking blood glucose prior to sleeping and during the night if possible. Again, personal experience is the best teacher. Help people experiment safely and learn from their experiences.

CONCLUSION

It is clear that many dietary components beyond the type and amount of carbohydrate affect glycemia. The consistent message is to educate people that fine-tuning glycemic control takes time and effort and is far from an exact science. It is critical that educators not convey the notion that glycemic control is easy, but rather that it is a daily challenge. Encourage people to keep records of their medication, food, activity, and blood glucose results on a chart such as those provided in Appendix III. It is only with the integration of all this information over time and with experience that people can learn what strategies and dosing techniques work best for them. Encourage pre- and postprandial monitoring so people can learn the impact of these various dietary components. Encourage people to experiment and learn.

CHAPTER ELEVEN

Impact on Glycemia of Non-Dietary Factors

In addition to nutrient intake and medications, many other factors can affect blood glucose control, including activity, illness, stress, travel, diabetic complications, and hormonal changes. This chapter covers guidelines for adjustments in carbohydrate intake related to these special situations and lifestyle changes.

PHYSICAL ACTIVITY AND EXERCISE

Regular physical activity is recommended for all people with diabetes who are healthy enough to exercise. The 2008 American Diabetes Association (ADA) recommendations for exercise are as follows:

- To improve glycemic control, reduce cardiovascular risk factors, contribute to weight loss, and improve well-being, people should perform at least 150 minutes per week of moderate-intensity aerobic physical activity (50–70% of maximum heart rate). The physical activity should be distributed over at least three days per week and with no more than two consecutive days without physical activity.
- In the absence of contraindications, people with type 2 diabetes should be encouraged to perform resistance exercise three times a week, targeting all major muscle groups, progressing in three sets of eight to ten repetitions at a weight that cannot be lifted more than eight to ten times (ADA 2008a).

Many factors influence the glycemic response to exercise, making it difficult to provide precise nutrition and medication guidelines that are applicable to everyone with diabetes (Franz 2002). Complicating matters, exercise can result in both hyperglycemia and hypoglycemia, frustrating nutrient and medicine recommendations. Frequent self-monitored blood glucose (SMBG) checks will help provide the basis for carbohydrate intake and insulin adjustments before, during, and after exercise.

Physical activity generally decreases blood glucose levels, as long as the person is not insulin deficient. However, when blood glucose is elevated >250 mg/dl with the presence of ketones and is not on the decline with active insulin on board, or when blood glucose is >300 mg/dl without ketosis, exercise can exacerbate hyperglycemia and should be avoided (Franz 2002).

Oral and other injectable diabetes medications that can cause hypoglycemia may need to be adjusted or omitted prior to or after exercise. People need to be advised accordingly by their prescribing health care provider. Refer to chapter 12 for specifics on blood glucose–lowering medications which can cause hypoglycemia.

Depending on the type, intensity, and duration of the activity, blood glucose levels can be lowered up to 36 hours after the activity and adjustments to carbohydrate intake may need to be considered. This decision should be based on:

- Pre-exercise blood glucose level
- Intensity of exercise
- Duration of exercise
- Time of day exercise in relation to insulin or diabetes medication peak action and duration
- Time of exercise in relation to most recent meal/snack
- Personal history of glycemic response to exercise
- Personal level of fitness

Advise people always to check their blood glucose levels prior to, during, and after exercise. Frequent post-exercise SMBG may be necessary, depending on the intensity and duration of the exercise (Colberg 2001). Record-keeping will help identify patterns and post-exercise glucose trends. Pattern management data will provide information to make necessary insulin or diabetes medication dose and carbohydrate intake adjustments.

If exercise occurs after a meal or snack, additional carbohydrate may not be necessary. If the activity is being performed more than two hours postprandially, a 15-gram carbohydrate snack is advised (Mullooly 2006). For more guidance, review Tables 11-1, 11-2, and 11-3.

Table 11-1. General Guidelines for Carbohydrate to Compensate for Exercise

Exercise Factor	Plan of Action
Pre-exercise blood glucose <100 mg/dl	Consume approx 15 grams of carbohydrate. If using CSII, consider using temporary decreased basal rate(s) and/or consider reduction of prior bolus dose if possible.
Unplanned or short in duration (<30 minutes)	Consume approx 15± grams of carbohydrate (insulin adjustment likely unnecessary).
Prolonged (>30 min) or intense (>60 minutes)	Consume 15 grams of carbohydrate every 30–60 minutes. Consider insulin dose reduction, 10–20%, and adjust per SMBG results.
Post-exercise	Consider insulin dose reduction (10–20% ±) and adjust per SMBG results. Additional carbohydrate may be necessary to reduce risk of hypoglycemia, as insulin sensitivity is increased and glycogen storage is enhanced (Bode 2004). Consider decreased ICR (less insulin is needed to cover carbohydrate, e.g., 1:20 instead of 1:15). Increase SMBG.

Table 11-2. Adjusting Preprandial Insulin for Activity

If the activity is to be performed 1–2 hours postprandial, advise people it may be necessary to lower the preprandial insulin dose to prevent hypoglycemia. Multiply the insulin dose by the factor below to determine the reduced preprandial insulin dose.

	Short Duration 15–30 minutes	Moderate Duration 31–60 minutes	Long Duration 1–2 hours
Low intensity	0.90	0.80	0.70
Moderate intensity	0.75	0.67	0.50
High intensity	0.67	0.50	0.33

Reprinted, by permission, from Scheiner 2006.

Table 11-3. Carbohydrate Needed Per Hour of Physical Activity

Snacks may be necessary for activities that take place before meals, are very intense, or last more than hour. The amount of carbohydrate needed depends on both the intensity of the activity and the person's size. The following table suggests the amount of carbohydrate grams needed per hour of activity. For 30 minutes of activity, suggest half the amounts listed.

	Weight				
	50 lb	100 lb	150 lb	200 lb	250 lb
Low intensity	5– 8 g	10–16 g	15–25 g	20–32 g	25–40 g
Moderate intensity	10–13 g	20–26 g	30–40 g	40–52 g	50–65 g
High intensity	15–18 g	30–36 g	45–55 g	60–72 g	75–90 g

Reprinted, by permission, from Scheiner 2006.

Fluid replacement is advisable if the physical activity is strenuous or lasts more than 60 minutes. If water is being consumed, additional carbohydrate can also be ingested in the form of a beverage. Drinks containing <8% carbohydrate empty from the stomach more rapidly than drinks containing a concentration of carbohydrate >10%. Fruit juices and most regular sodas contain about 12% carbohydrate and can lead to gastrointestinal upset, such as cramps, nausea, diarrhea, or bloating. This can be remedied by diluting the sports drink or beverage with water. However, since the carbohydrate in beverages is absorbed quickly, a few ounces must be consumed every five to ten minutes to provide the consistent supply of fuel required by the body's active muscles. This option also reduces the total calories consumed. In a beverage, 15 grams of carbohydrate contains 60 kcal, while 15 grams of carbohydrate in a food choice that includes protein or fat can total 150 calories (Mullooly 2006).

ILLNESS, SICK DAY MANAGEMENT, AND SURGERY

Illness, even short term or minor, can have adverse effects on blood glucose control. Colds, sore throats, mild infections, flu symptoms, nausea, vomiting, diarrhea, and fever can increase blood glucose. Even dental or minor outpatient surgery can impact diabetes management.

Flu-like symptoms often mimic the development of diabetic ketoacidosis and should not be ignored. People with type 2 diabetes rarely have ketones because they usually still have some endogenous insulin production. However, on sick days, counterregulatory hormones and catecholamines may trigger ketosis in people with type 2 diabetes as well as in those with type 1 diabetes. A general recommendation is for all people who have diabetes to check for ketones during illness (Hinnen and Guthrie 2005). Advise people to always have ketone testing supplies (urine and/or blood) available, and to check expiration dates routinely. Urine ketone test strips are available in individually foil-wrapped boxes as well as in vials. At present, several meters have the ability to check the blood ketone level (though this option is more costly than urine ketone check strips).

Every person with diabetes, both type 1 and type 2, should have carbohydrate replacement on hand, especially during the winter flu season. Encourage people to "stock up" and be prepared. Also provide guidelines to people so they know whom to contact and what to do for specific situations.

Sick day guidelines

In general, people who have diabetes should follow these guidelines during illness:

- Increase SMBG to detect and treat problems before they worsen.
- Start drinking non-caloric fluids one to two hours after any vomiting to prevent dehydration. Drink the fluids slowly. Non-caloric fluids include:
  - Water
  - Instant broth
  - Diet drinks
  - Sugar-free tea/coffee (may want to use decaffeinated)
  - Sugar-free ice pops
  - Sugar-free gelatin

- If unable to consume solids, replace carbohydrate with fluid equivalents. Consume 10–15 grams of carbohydrate every one to two hours. Substitutions include:
  - 1/2 cup fruit juice or fruit drink
  - 1/2 cup regular gelatin
  - 1/2–3/4 cup regular soda
  - One regular double ice pop
  - One fruit juice ice pop
  - 1/4 cup sherbet
  - 1 cup soup
  - 1 cup milk
  - 1/4 cup regular pudding
  - 1/2 cup sugar-free pudding
  - 1/2 cup ice cream

- When the person is able to tolerate solid food, suggest small, frequent amounts of food containing 10–15 grams of carbohydrate, including:
  - 1/2 cup cooked cereal
  - 1/2 cup mashed potatoes
  - 1/3 cup rice
  - One slice bread/toast
  - Three graham cracker halves
  - Six saltine crackers
  - Six vanilla wafers

Depending on the severity of the illness, symptoms, and blood glucose results, temporarily increased insulin dose adjustments will be necessary. Insulin doses should be increased gradually based on frequent SMBG and, if applicable, ketone test results. More frequent correction bolus doses may be necessary. With multiple daily injection (MDI) and continuous subcutaneous insulin infusion (CSII) therapy, meal doses can be calculated based on the person's actual intake, and be given postprandial to prevent hypoglycemia.

People who use oral agents and other injectable diabetes medications should be advised to contact their health care provider for specific medication adjustment guidelines.

STRESS

Stress, though a normal part of life, can cause some of the most erratic glycemic responses. Stressors can be positive and negative, short- or long-term, and can affect a person's ability to achieve and maintain good control. Inadequate sleep, too much food, inactivity, and the release of counterregulatory hormones can all increase blood glucose levels.

To prevent the onset of ketosis during times of stress, as with illness, people with type 1 diabetes should check for ketones when blood glucose is 250 mg/dl or higher and take appropriate action. Also similar to illness, insulin needs increase during stress. Eating patterns change, and many people consume excess food in response, increasing their need for additional insulin to cover the increase in caloric intake. Both basal and bolus insulin doses will need to be increased. Conversely, some people respond to stress by eating less or omitting meals, putting them at a potential risk for hypoglycemia.

People who use MDI or CSII therapy should be encouraged to perform frequent SMBG whenever they experience stress to identify their own pattern of blood glucose changes. Those who use CSII have the option of setting temporary increased or decreased basal rate settings for a specific number of hours to compensate for changes in their insulin requirements. Frequent SMBG is crucial during periods of stress and can help identify patterns of blood glucose control.

When stress is identified as a recurrent cause for changes in eating habits, weight, and medication, with accompanying deteriorating control, it is appropriate to consider referral to a mental health professional.

CHANGES IN ROUTINE AND DELAYED MEALS

Any change in routine or schedule can necessitate a change in insulin doses and/or carbohydrate counting methodologies. Increased activity, altered meal timing, and changes in the type and amounts of meals all require adjustments.

For changes in routine that result in periods of increased activity, such as on vacation, a 10–20% or more decrease in basal insulin doses may be necessary. Any insulin-to-carbohydrate ratio (ICR) and insulin correction factor (CF) may also need to change, as the body becomes more sensitive to insulin with the extra activity. Alter these numbers so that less insulin is used to cover carbohydrate, e.g., 1 unit to 20 grams instead of 1 unit to 15 grams.

Holidays and eating unfamiliar foods at unusual times may also necessitate additional changes and correction doses. In addition to changes in the timing and amounts of bolus insulin needed to cover larger or longer meals, delayed meals may require consuming a modest (15–30 grams) amount of carbohydrate to prevent hypoglycemia. Teach people to be prepared with a readily available carbohydrate at hand. Experience is the best teacher—encourage people to "learn from the last time" by keeping good records and making adjustments based on patterns.

TRAVEL

In contemporary society, travel may be part of an exciting vacation or simply a routine part of a day-to-day job. Whatever the reason, travel often involves drastic departures from routine meal plans and activity levels. Eating new and/or unfamiliar foods and enjoying increased activity can be fun, but may present some challenges. These challenges are often exacerbated by time zone changes.

Whether travel is for business or pleasure, teach people to be prepared for delays, missed meals, and interrupted plans. Carbohydrate sources should be readily available in carry-on (depending on current airline regulations) or close-at-hand luggage. Suggested items to carry include:

- Small can or box of fruit juice
- Dried fruit, e.g., raisins
- Fruit roll-ups
- Crackers
- Granola bars
- Gingersnaps or vanilla wafers

Travel and unfamiliar customs can result in meal delays. In general, advise people to wait until their meal is in front of them before taking their mealtime bolus insulin or injectable or oral diabetes medication. If insulin or other diabetes medication has already been taken, it may be necessary to consume a small amount (10–15 grams) of carbohydrate before the meal is served.

Time zone changes

Traveling east means the day is shorter and less insulin may be needed. Decrease the basal dose of insulin 10–30% depending on the number of time zone changes. If traveling across mainland United States, the time change is only 3 hours, and minimal, if any, adjustment in the basal dose will be necessary. Travel from Alaska or Hawaii across mainland United States and international eastbound travel require a greater change.

Westbound travel increases the hours in a day, creating a need for additional insulin to cover the extra hours. This may entail an increase in the total basal dose, or splitting the basal dose. Meal bolus insulin will cover any additional food intake. Domestic and international westbound travel necessitates more insulin, both basal and bolus doses.

Prolonged plane, train, or automobile travel may also necessitate a higher basal insulin dose, independent of time zone changes. This is especially true for people whose activity level is lower than usual during their travel time. A higher altitude may result in an increased need for insulin (Walsh and Roberts 2006). It is best to make changes by 5–10%; trial-and-error and record keeping will help people determine appropriate dose changes.

Travel does not usually necessitate a change in ICR(s), unless the person has a higher ratio in the morning. However, a change in time zones may require a change in ICR for the meal that would occur during the usual time of day. And mealtimes are different in other countries. Some cultures have their main meal in the middle of the day, others later in the evening than the traditional American culture, so mealtime insulin doses will need adjustments as well to better match the person's intake.

People who use CSII can make time zone adjustments easily. If the person's basal rates vary only slightly, he or she can set the pump clock to the time zone of the destination during the course of the journey or upon arrival. If the basal rates vary dramatically over 24 hours, it's best to make gradual changes in steps by 1 1/2 hours each day. A six-hour time zone change, for example, would be adjusted over 4 days with 1 1/2-hour adjustments each day (Wolpert 2002).

People with type 2 diabetes who take oral or other injectable diabetes medications should check with their health care provider for specific medication adjustment guidelines for travel that involves changes in time zones.

GASTROPARESIS

Gastroparesis is a form of autonomic neuropathy that results in erratic or delayed digestion. It is believed that gastroparesis develops in up to 50% of people with diabetes (Feigenbaum 2006). The most common cause of this condition is damage to the vagus nerve. However, research indicates that people with diabetes have variable rates of gastric emptying, ranging from accelerated gastric emptying without any symptoms of gastrointestinal dysfunction (Nowak et al. 1995) to life-disturbing and burdensome manifestations.

The symptoms associated with gastroparesis include heartburn, reflux of foods and liquids into the esophagus, dysphagia, anorexia, nausea, vomiting, early satiety, and postprandial bloating and fullness. Delayed nutrient absorption can complicate blood glucose control, producing erratic swings between postprandial hypoglycemia and severe hyperglycemia.

People who have gastroparesis are sometimes deficient in vitamins B12 and D and iron and may require supplementation. Meals should be low in fiber and fat content and small in volume. Six smaller meals throughout the day may be better tolerated than three large meals. It may also be necessary to puree or liquefy foods. Hypoglycemia treatment should consist of carbohydrate sources that are absorbed in the mouth, such as liquids, gels, and hard candies.

Gastroparesis requires frequent SMBG. Increased postprandial checks are most helpful in determining how to adjust food intake and the timing and dose of mealtime bolus insulin. It is often suggested to delay the rapid-acting insulin meal bolus until after the meal has been consumed. The meal bolus could then be administered when the blood glucose level begins to rise. Another option is to use short-acting (regular) insulin in place of rapid-acting insulin analogs. People who use CSII can program an extended or combination meal bolus to accommodate their needs. Pump users who have gastroparesis can also increase their daytime (i.e., mealtime) basal rate(s), perhaps as high as 70% of their total daily dose, along with reduced boluses (Walsh and Roberts 2006). Trial and error and detailed record keeping will help determine percentages of the bolus to be delivered immediately or over time.

MENSES AND HORMONAL CHANGES

Some women notice that their sensitivity to insulin changes at different times during their menstrual cycle (Case and Reid 1998; Moberg et al. 1995). Not only will basal insulin dose adjustments be necessary, but some women may need to change their ICR(s) and CF(s) as well. Increased episodes of hypoglycemia and hyperglycemia tend to occur more often, with the latter a result of both hormonal changes and increases in cravings for high-carbohydrate foods during the premenstrual phase (Homko 2005).

It is common for many women to notice hyperglycemia for a few days prior to their menstrual period. Some women require large increases in their total insulin needs, while others may require only small adjustments. Insulin requirements may also change during ovulation. Most women tend to develop their own monthly pattern of insulin requirements, and these requirements remain fairly consistent month-to-month. Women whose cycles are irregular will have less consistent patterns of insulin requirements.

Both basal insulin and bolus insulin doses may need to be adjusted, as well as CFs. If using CSII, an alternate basal pattern specific to monthly or hormonal changes can be programmed. Trial and error and detailed record-keeping will help determine appropriate insulin requirements to achieve and maintain blood glucose control.

Women who are perimenopausal and those who are in menopause will also experience hormonal fluctuations (Dougherty and Pastors 2007) and may require changes in their insulin doses. Detailed record-keeping to identify trends and patterns will assist in the determination of appropriate adjustments.

CONCLUSION

Many people are surprised to find that so many non-dietary factors play a dominant role in blood glucose control, and that tight glycemic control can often be difficult and confusing. It's important to stress that with all of the factors that can influence glycemic responses, perfect control might not be possible. However, teach that it's best to be cognizant of the many variables that can affect blood glucose control and reinforce the need to plan for them as best as one can.

CHAPTER TWELVE

Blood Glucose– Lowering and Related Medications

UNDERSTANDING NORMAL INSULIN RESPONSE

In normal human physiology, there is continuous secretion of a small amount of insulin at a relatively constant level 24 hours per day. This basal insulin maintains glycemia in a narrow range, with fasting normoglycemia between 70 and 100 mg/dl and postprandial glycemia at or below 140 mg/dl (Aronoff et al. 2004). Basal insulin manages hepatic glucose output and glucose disposal in the fasting state. Insulin secretion is glucose-dependent and insulin is not secreted when blood glucose concentrations fall below 60 mg/dl. When blood glucose levels increase above 60 mg/dl, people who do not have diabetes secrete insulin in increasing amounts (Wallum et al. 1992). Amylin is also co-secreted by the pancreatic β-cells and glucagon is secreted from the pancreatic alpha cells, both in response to nutrient intake.

With the ingestion of food, the body secretes insulin in precise amounts to match the rise in glucose from nutrient intake to stimulate glucose utilization and storage while inhibiting hepatic glucose output. The secretion of bolus insulin establishes and helps maintain postprandial euglycemia. Figure 12-1 illustrates the nondiabetic release of basal and bolus insulin.

Bolus insulin is secreted in two phases, detailed in Figure 12-2. First-phase insulin release occurs within 15 minutes of initial food consumption and the subsequent rise of blood glucose. During the first phase, the pancreas secretes a small burst of insulin that has previously been produced and is waiting in the pancreas to be used. Second-phase insulin release is more gradual and occurs over the next 120–180 minutes. This insulin is newly produced, with the amount released matching the rise in blood glucose from consumed carbohydrate.

Figure 12-1. Physiologic Insulin Secretion

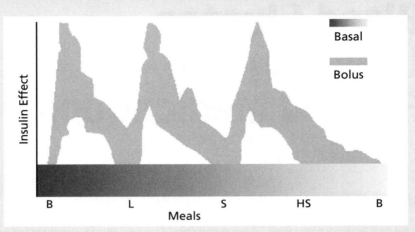

Reprinted, by permission, from Childs and Kruger 2005.

Figure 12-2. Normal Insulin Release for Food

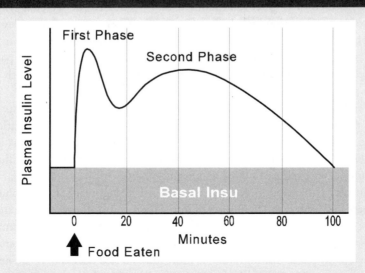

Reprinted, by permission, from Walsh and Roberts 2006.

Insulin is necessary for the metabolism of macronutrients (carbohydrate, protein, and fat) as well as for the management of hepatic glucose production. Without insulin, blood glucose concentrations increase to dangerous and potentially life-threatening levels. People with type 1 diabetes do not produce insulin—their pancreatic ß-cells are compromised and exogenous insulin is necessary for survival. In people with type 2 diabetes, there is insulin deficiency and/or insulin resistance.

Both basal and bolus insulin therapies are necessary for those with type 1 diabetes, and to be most effective, should closely mimic normal insulin physiology. People with type 2 diabetes may require insulin in the later stages of the progression of their disease. The insulin may be supplemental to oral (single- or multiple-agent) therapy, or insulin therapy alone may be used to effectively manage type 2 diabetes.

INSULIN REGIMENS

Insulin regimens vary and should be designed with the person's lifestyle in mind. Factors taken into consideration include meal/snack schedule, work or activity schedule, sleeping habits, medications, and personal (emotional) factors (Childs and Kruger 2005).

Basal-bolus insulin therapy

There are many different approaches to insulin therapy, ranging from conventional regimens of one to two daily injections to intensive therapies of multiple daily injections (MDI) or continuous subcutaneous insulin infusion (CSII) therapy. Refer to chapter 7 for more details.

Basal insulin

In MDI therapy, intermediate- or long-acting (basal) insulin maintains diurnal normoglycemia between meals as well as nocturnal normoglycemia by reducing hepatic glucose production. Basal insulin constitutes about 50% of the total daily dose (TDD) (Skyler 2004), but can range from 45–60%, and is given either once daily or split between two doses. Intermediate-acting and long-acting insulins can be considered basal insulins.

With CSII, an insulin pump releases individualized programmed amounts of rapid-acting insulin continuously in very small doses to create basal insulin.

Bolus insulin

In conventional insulin therapy (not MDI or CSII), bolus insulin may be in the form of one or two fixed daily doses of rapid- or short-acting insulin taken or manually user-mixed with intermediate- or long-acting insulin. The rapid- or short-acting insulin may also be purchased premixed with intermediate-acting insulin. Whether injected separately, injected from a premixed pen, drawn from two separate vials and mixed by the person, or drawn from a premixed vial, this fixed-dose regimen is referred to as a split-mixed regimen. Currently, a rapid- or short-acting insulin or insulin analog cannot be mixed in the same syringe or pen with a long-acting insulin analog due to differences in pH.

While conventional insulin therapy consists of one or two daily insulin injections, intensive therapy includes individualized dose-adjusted multiple injections of bolus insulin with a fixed basal regimen. MDI and CSII therapy are both considered intensive therapy. Using these intensive therapies, bolus doses are created and administered to match nutrient intake and correct out-of-range glycemia.

INSULIN PHARMACOKINETICS AND PHARMACODYNAMICS

The "action curves" of insulins in medical literature and product information show the insulin concentration in the blood over a time period (pharmacokinetics). This is not, however, a direct measure of insulin action in the control of blood glucose levels (pharmacodynamics). Figure 12-3 illustrates these differences. In blood glucose control, the pharmacodynamics are most pertinent, however, the pharmacokinetic action curves are most often used by health care providers.

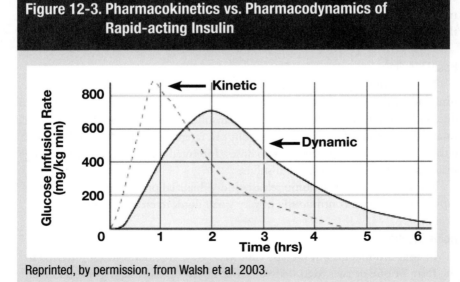

Figure 12-3. Pharmacokinetics vs. Pharmacodynamics of Rapid-acting Insulin

Reprinted, by permission, from Walsh et al. 2003.

Research studies have compared doses of insulin lispro and insulin aspart to regular insulin. One study showed that the mean (+ SD) peak action of insulin lispro was 99 + 39 minutes (span of 60–138 minutes) (Howey et al. 1994). Another study showed that the mean (+ SD) peak action of insulin aspart was 94 + 46 minutes (span of 48–140 minutes) (Mudaliar et al. 1999). It is important to note that appreciation of this lag time is critical in the control of postprandial hyperglycemia (Hirsch 2005). Additional research demonstrates that with a preprandial blood glucose of 180 mg/dl, postprandial hyperglycemia is minimized when the lag time (amount of time before the meal insulin is taken) is at least 15 minutes, and that longer lag times are more desirable when there is more profound hyperglycemia (Hirsch 2005).

Additional research has revealed that a dose of insulin aspart still had significant activity at 300 minutes. At three hours after the injection of 10 units of insulin, 40% of this dose (4 units) of insulin aspart still remained active (Hirsch 2005). Other research indicates that rapid-acting insulin has a longer action curve than the four to five hours depicted in Figure 12-3, and some clinicians believe

About Pre-Mixed Insulin

Premixed insulins, combinations of rapid- or short-acting insulin and intermediate-acting insulin, offer the convenience and ease of a single injection without the challenge of drawing two insulins from two separate vials into one syringe. These insulins are often the insulin of choice for the person who may be visually impaired or who has dexterity problems. However, premixed and fixed-mixed insulin doses do not permit variations in carbohydrate intake and do not offer the freedom and flexibility of basal-bolus regimens, especially for those with type 1 diabetes.

For those with type 2 diabetes, especially in the earlier years of their disease when they have some endogenous insulin production, the advantages of basal-bolus therapy in improving A1C control can be difficult to discern (Braithwaite 2005). However, the use of peakless insulin (insulin glargine and insulin detemir) in comparison to NPH during prandial use of short-acting insulin and the use of a rapid-acting analog insulin in comparison to short-acting insulin during MDI therapy have been shown to produce less hypoglycemia and to reduce postprandial hyperglycemia (Rosetti et al. 2003; Rosenstock et al. 2001). The necessity to deal with repeated episodes of hyperglycemia and hypoglycemia during premixed or fixed-dose therapy, without any clear comprehension of what each dose of insulin in a split-mixed regimen achieves, is not easy for the person with diabetes (Braithwaite 2005). Advanced Carbohydrate Counting skills and the use of an individual insulin-to-carbohydrate ratio (ICR) in intensive therapy afford more flexibility in one's lifestyle (DAFNE Study Group 2002).

that 20–25% of a dose of insulin lispro or insulin aspart will be used each hour after it has been injected (Walsh and Roberts 2006).

The variability in insulin pharmacodynamics between individuals who have diabetes and even within the same person from day to day must also be recognized. From a practical standpoint, this means that insulin action curves should be a framework, not steadfast rules, for educators and people with diabetes. People need to perform SMBG checks at various times of the day over several days to obtain a sense of their body's individual response to various insulins. And there will also be variation depending on a myriad of factors.

EXAMPLES OF INSULIN REGIMENS

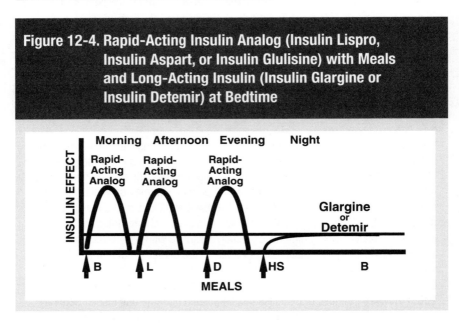

Figure 12-4. Rapid-Acting Insulin Analog (Insulin Lispro, Insulin Aspart, or Insulin Glulisine) with Meals and Long-Acting Insulin (Insulin Glargine or Insulin Detemir) at Bedtime

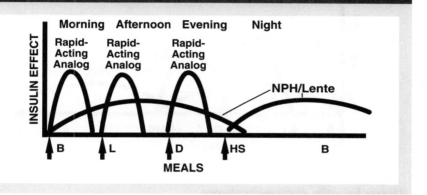

Figure 12-5. Rapid-Acting Insulin Analog (Insulin Lispro, Insulin Aspart, or Insulin Glulisine) with Meals and Intermediate-Acting Insulin (NPH/Lente) Before Breakfast and at Bedtime

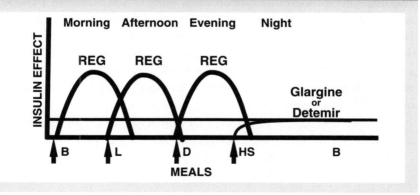

Figure 12-6. Short-Acting (Regular) Insulin with Meals and Long-Acting (Insulin Glargine or Insulin Detemir) at Bedtime

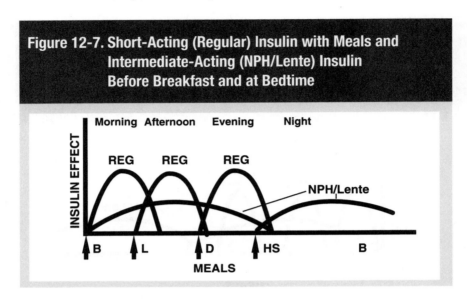

Figure 12-7. Short-Acting (Regular) Insulin with Meals and Intermediate-Acting (NPH/Lente) Insulin Before Breakfast and at Bedtime

About insulin concentrations

Through the years, there have also been modifications in insulin concentrations. The U-40 and U-80 insulins, while still available in other countries (ADA 2003), have been replaced in the United States with U-100 insulin. Other insulin concentrations, such as U-400, used in implantable pumps, and U-500 are also available. One must exercise caution when using U-500 insulin in a U-100 insulin syringe, as the concentration of U-500 insulin is five times the potency of U-100 insulin. U-500 insulin may be preferred by those who require large single doses (>100 units) of U-100 insulin. ICRs are not affected by different insulin concentrations, but the dosage drawn from a different concentration is markedly different. The amount of U-500 insulin drawn in a U-100 insulin syringe would be one-fifth the amount.

> **Example:** If the carbohydrate bolus for an ICR of 1:15 is 5 units of U-100 insulin (for 60 grams of carbohydrate), the amount of U-500 insulin drawn in a U-100 syringe would be only 1 unit, as the U-500 insulin is 5 times the concentration of U-100 insulin.

OTHER INJECTABLE MEDICATIONS

In 2005, the U.S. FDA approved two new injectable first-in-class diabetes medications: Pramlintide acetate injection, an amylinomimetic, or amylin analog (for people with type 1 or type 2 diabetes who take mealtime insulin), and exenatide injection, an incretin mimetic (for patients with type 2 diabetes).

Amylinomimetics

Until fairly recently, insulin was the only pancreatic ß-cell hormone known to affect blood glucose. However, in 1987 it was discovered that amylin, a neuroendocrine hormone, is co-secreted with insulin by the ß-cells of the pancreas. Like insulin, it works in response to food consumption, but, unlike insulin, does not stimulate glucose uptake from the blood into tissue cells. Amylin instead regulates gastric emptying, induces satiety, and contributes to the suppression of glucagon in the postprandial state (Aronoff et al. 2004; Kruger and Gloster 2004). Amylin is deficient in people with type 1 diabetes and diminished in people with type 2 diabetes.

A synthetic analog of amylin, pramlintide, has been developed to use in conjunction with mealtime insulin for both those with type 1 and type 2 diabetes (including those with type 2 diabetes who may also be using a sulfonylurea or metformin). Pramlintide therapy suppresses inappropriate postprandial glucagon secretion and slows gastric emptying, thereby improving postprandial glucose and minimizing glucose fluctuations. It also creates satiety, a feeling of fullness, which results in less food intake and weight loss (Weyer et al. 2001). Pramlintide is injected three times daily at the start of a meal containing at least 250 kcal or 30 grams of carbohydrate and is adjusted over several weeks to its maintenance dose. Mealtime (bolus) insulin should be reduced 50% at the initiation of pramlintide therapy to reduce the risk of insulin-induced severe hypoglycemia (Karl 2006), and then adjusted to its maintenance dose. Basal insulin may also need to be adjusted in people who lose weight.

Incretin mimetics

In the 1960s, it was learned that ingested food caused a more potent release of insulin than intravenously infused glucose (Perley and Kipnis 1967), which made it apparent that hormones in addition to insulin affect glycemia. This became known as the "incretin effect" and started the search for gut hormones that play a role in the hormonal regulation of glucose disappearance. Several incretin hormones, including gastric inhibitory polypeptide (GIP) and glucagon-like peptide-1 (GLP-1), have been identified. GLP-1 is secreted in greater concentrations and has become well characterized for its role in glucose metabolism. GLP-1 is synthesized and secreted by the L-cells of the ileum and colon. It stimulates insulin secretion in a glucose-dependent manner, inhibits glucagon secretion, and slows gastric emptying (Kruger 2006). GLP-1 is significantly reduced postprandially in people with type 2 diabetes or those with impaired glucose tolerance (Nauck et al. 1993).

Exenatide is a synthetic GLP-1 receptor agonist (Riddle and Drucker 2006).

Exenatide is for use in type 2 diabetes as adjunctive therapy with metformin, a sulfonylurea, a thiazolidinedione (TZD), a combination of a sulfonylurea and metformin, or a TZD and metformin (BYETTA 2007). Studies have shown that exenatide enhances glucose-dependent insulin secretion from pancreatic β-cells, restores first-phase insulin response, and suppresses glucagon secretion from pancreatic alpha cells during hyperglycemia, which leads to enhanced insulin response to food, a reduction of glucose output from the liver, reduced food intake (which results in weight loss), and slowed gastric emptying, allowing for timely absorption of nutrients. Exenatide improves postprandial and fasting glucose, lowers A1C, and promotes weight loss (BYETTA 2007). Exenatide is injected twice daily at a minimum of six hours apart before any two main meals of the day, regardless of specific caloric or carbohydrate intake.

ORAL DIABETES MEDICATIONS

During the 1940s, around the time of World War II, it was noticed that antibacterial agents (sulfa drugs) seemed to lower blood glucose. But it wasn't until the 1950s that this discovery led to the introduction in the United States of sulfa-like drugs for the treatment of diabetes. The late 1950s saw the introduction of the first class of diabetes anti-hypoglycemic oral medication in the form of first-generation sulfonylureas. Second-generation sulfonylureas appeared in the 1970s. Through the last forty years, five additional drug classes for orally administered agents for type 2 diabetes have been introduced, and another class of oral diabetes medications was recently added in 2006. Currently, type 2 diabetes oral drug classes include (see Appendix II for more on blood glucose–lowering medications):

- Sulfonylureas
- Meglitinides
- Biguanides
- Thiazolidinediones (TZDs)
- Alpha-glucosidase inhibitors
- DPP-IV (dipeptidyl peptidase 4) inhibitors, also called incretin enhancers

While Advanced Carbohydrate Counting is best suited for intensive insulin therapies such as MDI and CSII, carbohydrate counting in general plays a role in the efficacy of oral diabetes medications as well. Some things to consider based on drug class:

- **Sulfonylureas:** Carbohydrate intake should be consistent day-to-day at meals and snacks. Can cause hypoglycemia and weight gain.

- **Meglitinides:** Best if carbohydrate intake is consistent day-to-day at meals and snacks, but the medication can be adjusted for the amount of carbohydrate to be consumed. Can cause hypoglycemia with decreased amount or absence of food.
- **Biguanides:** Best if carbohydrate intake is consistent day-to-day at meals and snacks. Does not cause hypoglycemia when used alone. Not for use in people who consume alcohol daily.
- **Thiazolidinediones (TZDs):** Best if carbohydrate intake is consistent day-to-day at meals and snacks. Does not cause hypoglycemia when used alone. Can cause weight gain.
- **Alpha-glucosidase inhibitors:** Best if carbohydrate intake is consistent day-to-day at meals and snacks. Slows down the breakdown of carbohydrate. Does not cause hypoglycemia when used alone, but hypoglycemia can occur with concomitant use of insulin or sulfonylurea. Treat hypoglycemia with glucose, not with complex carbohydrate, due to the action of the medication.
- **DPP-IV (dipeptidyl peptidase 4) inhibitors:** Best if carbohydrate intake is consistent day-to-day at meals and snacks. Does not cause hypoglycemia.

Single medication combinations of drugs from two classes are also approved and widely used. There are currently four combination drug class medications:

- Biguanide with DPP-IV inhibitor
- Biguanide with sulfonylurea
- Biguanide with TZD
- TZD with sulfonylurea

Today, the management of type 2 diabetes includes oral therapy with one medication, oral combination therapy, and/or oral/injectable therapy. Numerous combinations of oral and injectable therapies can be used safely (Steil 2006):

- Sulfonylurea and alpha-glucosidase inhibitor
- Sulfonylurea and amylinomimetic (pramlintide)
- Sulfonylurea and biguanide (metformin)
- Sulfonylurea and DPP-IV inhibitor
- Sulfonylurea and incretin mimetic (exenatide)
- Sulfonylurea and TZD
- Biguanide (metformin) and amylinomimetic (pramlintide)
- Biguanide (metformin) and incretin mimetic (exenatide)
- Biguanide (metformin) and meglitinide
- Biguanide (metformin) and TZD
- TZD and incretin mimetic (exenatide) (BYETTA 2007)

- TZD and meglitinide
- DPP-IV and biguanide (metformin)
- DPP-IV and TZD

CONCLUSION

The addition of new drug classes and insulin analogs provides both benefits and challenges for persons with diabetes as well as for the clinicians who help them manage their diabetes. Medical nutrition therapy, specifically carbohydrate counting, is an integral component in the management of diabetes and can play a role in the use of various pharmacologic diabetes therapies.

CHAPTER THIRTEEN

Process to Develop and Maintain Personal Carbohydrate Counts

As this book has illustrated, a number of factors contribute to proper carbohydrate counting, and subsequently, good glycemic control. However, two key factors often determine a person's success with carbohydrate counting, whether Basic or Advanced:

1. A willingness and ability to determine carbohydrate counts of the foods they eat

2. Consistent weighing and measuring of foods to assure proper servings

Without these two factors, it is difficult to properly count carbohydrates. Fortunately, there are a number of resources available to simplify the process. Educators point people to Nutrition Facts panels, discuss consistent weighing and measuring of foods, and encourage use of food databases that contain the carbohydrate counts for thousands of foods in books, online, or in an insulin pump.

While it's fortunate that these resources exist, their ubiquity can also make the task of assessing carbohydrate counts seem and be overwhelming. Educators may want to use another approach: take advantage of the fact that people are creatures of habit regarding their food choices and that, day to day, people eat a relatively narrow array of foods. They commonly purchase similar foods, put together similar meals and snacks, and even order similar items at their favorite restaurants.

Using this premise, help people realize that if they obtain the carbohydrate counts for the narrow list of foods they regularly consume, they will have much of the information they need for many of their meals. With their "personal carbohydrate counts" in hand, they can minimize the energy and effort of carbohydrate counting while they increase their accuracy. The following provides a step-by-step process for teaching people to build and maintain their personal carbohydrate counts, which can then be used for either Basic or Advanced Carbohydrate Counting.

PERSONAL CARBOHYDRATE COUNTS

1. Brainstorm a list of 50–100 commonly eaten foods on a form, such as the sample in Table 13-1. Encourage people to observe the foods in their refrigerator, pantry, and freezer. Encourage them to think about the foods they regularly eat for breakfast, lunch, dinner, and snacks.

2. Next to each of the foods recorded in Step #1, record the amount of each food that is commonly eaten under "Amount I Eat" in Table 13-1. Encourage people to obtain these amounts by weighing and measuring foods over a few weeks as they eat them. For example, as the person prepares breakfast and pours dry cereal into the commonly used serving item, do one more step: pour the cereal into a measuring cup. Record the amount in the chart. To estimate the weights of fruits, weigh a few apples, bananas, and oranges. Get an average weight and record it. Measure the amount of mashed potatoes, rice, and other commonly eaten foods.

3. To complete the last column in Table 13-1, encourage people to determine the carbohydrate counts of these foods in the amounts they commonly eat. Encourage them to use the carbohydrate counting resources noted in Appendix I. Do remind them that if a Nutrition Facts panel is available for a given food, they should use it. This is likely the most accurate information because it is product and brand specific; it's also easy to obtain. Remind people to make sure the information they record is for the serving they eat, not the food label serving (if they are not the same).

4. After they have completed Table 13-1 and obtained the carbohydrate counts for the foods that they regularly eat, encourage people to determine the total carbohydrate count for common meals they eat. People commonly eat the same combination of foods at meals and snacks day after day, and often have one of three choices they eat at breakfast and lunch. Dinner is a meal that often varies more than the others. Table 13-2 is a form that can be used for this step.

Once these two tables are completed, people can use this information to ascertain the carbohydrate counts of individual foods and carbohydrate counts of common meals utilizing carbohydrate counting resources in Appendix I. Encourage people to develop and maintain these charts in a way that works best for them. Some people may want to put them on small index cards they can carry in their diabetes supplies, others may want to laminate the cards. Some may want to avoid cards and keep this information in a personal digital assistant, smart phone, or other high-tech device. No matter the method, encourage people to keep up the database and add foods and meals over time as appropriate.

Table 13-1. Sample Personal Food Database

Food	Amount I Eat	Carbohydrate Count (grams)
Bran Flakes	3/4 cup	23
Honey Nut Cheerios	3/4 cup	17
Milk, fat free	1 1/4 cup	15
Banana	1 small	21
Apple, Granny Smith	1 small (6 ounce)	23
Whole-wheat bread—Arnold	1 slice	18
American cheese slices—2% milk	1 slice	2
Tomato soup—Campbell's	1 can (8-ounce), prepared with 1 container of fat-free milk	31

Table 13-2. Carbohydrate Counts of Common Meals and Snacks

Meals	Amount I Eat	Carbohydrate Count (grams)
Breakfast #1		
Bran Flakes	3/4 cup	23
Honey Nut Cheerios	3/4 cup	17
Milk, fat free	1 1/4 cup	15
Banana	1 small	21
	Total	76
Breakfast #2		
Whole wheat bread – Arnold	2 slices	36
American cheese slices	2 slices	2
Apple	1 medium	23
	Total	61

INTEGRATION OF PERSONAL CARBOHYDRATE COUNTS WITH INSULIN PUMPS

The above process can and should be integrated into continuous subcutaneous insulin infusion (CSII) therapy to increase the accuracy of carbohydrate counts. Several of today's insulin pumps can deliver precise bolus doses calculated out to two decimal points. It is important that this level of precision in insulin dosing be meshed with accuracy of carbohydrate counts. Otherwise the value of precise insulin dosing is minimized.

Today's insulin pumps vary in their availability of integrated food databases. Some pumps contain no food database, some contain a static database that simply provides some nutrition information for commonly eaten foods, and others provide a customizable food database in which a person can add or delete foods and related nutrient information. The latter type of database then allows a person to use the carbohydrate counts of foods and/or meals (the carbohydrate counts of several foods added together) to determine a carbohydrate count and a matched bolus insulin dose based on an individualized insulin-to-carbohydrate ratio (ICR).

To help people who use an insulin pump that contains a food database that interfaces with their dosing capabilities, encourage them to customize the food database as much as possible using a process similar to the one above. With their pump food database, encourage them to delete foods they will never eat and/or create a custom database within the pump's software and the pump itself. The fewer foods people need to scroll through and the more they delete foods they'll never eat, the more likely they are to find their customized database helpful and easy to use. In addition, several pumps provide people with the option of maintaining the carbohydrate counts of meals that they regularly eat. Then it's the press of a few buttons to get the carbohydrate count for these meals and an accurate dose.

CONCLUSION

Accurate carbohydrate counting remains a critical piece of achieving good blood glucose control. The more educators can help people count their carbohydrate intake accurately, the more likely people are to achieve their blood glucose targets.

Appendices

Resources for Carbohydrate Counting and Insulin Pump Therapy

People need to be provided with reliable, accessible, and useful carbohydrate-counting resources. It is not necessary to inundate people with choices. Recommend resources based on a person's eating habits and food choices, as well as the format of resources they are likely to use (e.g., book or online). Then suggest the key resources to fit their needs.

BOOKS THAT TEACH CARBOHYDRATE COUNTING

- Warshaw, H.W., K. Kulkarni. 2004. *The American Diabetes Association Complete Guide to Carb Counting,* 2nd edition. Alexandria, VA: American Diabetes Association.*

- Daly, A., K. Bolderman, M. Franz, K. Kulkarni. 2003. *Basic Carbohydrate Counting.* Alexandria, VA: American Diabetes Association; Chicago: American Dietetic Association.*

- Daly, A., K. Bolderman, M. Franz, K. Kulkarni. 2003. *Advanced Carbohydrate Counting.* Alexandria, VA: American Diabetes Association; Chicago: American Dietetic Association.*

- Scheiner, G. 2006. *The Ultimate Guide to Accurate Carb Counting.* Emeryville, CA: Marlowe Diabetes Library.

---

*Order these books from 800-ADA-ORDER (232-6733) or at *www.diabetes.org*

BOOKS AND PRINT MATERIAL WITH CARBOHYDRATE COUNTS

Keep in mind that the primary resource for carbohydrate information, if it is available, should be the Nutrition Facts panel of food labels (see chapter 4).

- Holzmeister, L. 2006. *The Diabetes Carbohydrate and Fat Gram Guide,* 3rd edition. Alexandria, VA: American Diabetes Association.*

- Borushek, A. 2006. *The Doctor's Pocket Calorie, Fat and Carbohydrates Counter. n.p.:* Family Health Publications.

- Kraus, B. 2005. *Barbara Kraus' Calories and Carbohydrates,* 16th edition. New York: Signet.
  This book provides the carbohydrate and calorie count for more than 8,000 foods, including fruits, vegetables, and other produce; meats, poultry, and seafood; desserts; many foods you know by their brand name; frozen entrees; and more.

- Netzer, C.T. 1998. *The Corinne T. Netzer Carbohydrate Counter,* 2nd edition. New York: Dell Publishing.
  This 486-page book provides the carbohydrate count for thousands of foods, including fruits, vegetables, and other produce; meats, poultry, and seafood; desserts; many foods you know by their brand name; frozen entrees; and more.

- Warshaw, H.S. 2005. *Guide to Healthy Restaurant Eating,* 3rd edition. Alexandria, VA: American Diabetes Association.
  This 700-page guide provides the basics about today's diabetes nutrition and meal planning goals, and strategies for healthy restaurant eating. Plus, there's nutrition information including carbohydrate, calories, fat, percent of calories as fat, saturated fat, cholesterol, sodium, fiber, and protein with servings or exchanges for nearly 5,000 menu items from more than 60 major restaurant chains.*

- Warshaw, H.S. 2006. *Guide to Healthy Fast Food Eating.* Alexandria, VA: American Diabetes Association.
  Nutrition information including carbohydrate, calories, fat, percent of calories as fat, saturated fat, cholesterol, sodium, fiber, and protein with servings or exchanges for about 1,500 menu items from the 13 major fast food chains.*

*Order these books from 800-ADA-ORDER (232-6733) or at *www.diabetes.org*

- Franklin Publishing, Inc. 2007. *Nutrition in the Fast Lane.* Indianapolis: Franklin Publishing, Inc.

    To purchase, call 1-800-634-1993 or visit *www.fastfoodfacts.com*. This booklet, which is updated annually, provides the nutrition information for 54 of the popular chain restaurants.

Note: Several insulin pumps come with external and internal software that contains a food database. Learn more about these and how to educate people about their suggested use in chapters 7 and 13.

SOFTWARE AND ONLINE RESOURCES FOR CARBOHYDRATE COUNTS

Note that some software allows people to track their nutrient intake, while some websites provide an option to download data to a computer, PDA, iPod, or other device. All websites were last accessed April 2008.

Websites

- *www.ars.usda.gov/ba/bhnrc/ndl*

    This is the U.S. federal government's nutrient database, which is searchable. It contains extensive nutrition information for about 7,000 basic foods. People can use this information at no cost. This database can be downloaded to a computer or PDA.

- *www.mypyramidtracker.gov*

    The online dietary assessment provides information on diet quality, related nutrition messages, and links to nutrient information. After providing a day's worth of dietary information, one will receive an overall evaluation by comparing the amounts of food consumed to current nutritional guidance. To give a better understanding of a diet over time, one can track what's eaten for up to a year.

- *www.calorieking.com*

- *www.betterbyte.red-deer.com/kdiet.htm*
    Kathleen's Diet Planner

- *www.myfooddiary.com*

- *www.nutritiondata.com*

- *www.dietfacts.com*

- *www.dwlz.com*

  Dottie's Weight Loss Zone is a combination of information provided directly by the restaurants or information obtained by people and provided to the website. Weight Watchers' points are included for many items.

- *www.healthydiningfinder.com*

  Joint venture between Healthy Dining and the National Restaurant Association.

- *www.chowbaby.com/fastfood/fast_food_nutrition.asp*

  Find nutrition information for large national and regional chain restaurants, from fast food to some sit-down American and ethnic fare.

Online restaurant information

The websites of many large chain restaurants provide basic nutrition information, including carbohydrate and fiber. This is valuable information for people who eat at these restaurants. It can also be used to educate people and illustrate the carbohydrate and calorie counts of restaurant foods.

Advanced software and websites

Below are software and websites available online that contain one or more of the following: carbohydrate counts of foods and ability to track intake; tracking of blood glucose results by meter download; integration and analysis of data; or the ability to communicate about data online with a health care provider.

- *www.dia-log.com*

  This site provides tracking logs and an ability to download results from blood glucose meters. For food and carbohydrate tracking, it links with www.myfooddairy.com

- *www.animascorp.com*
  EZManager Plus from Animas Corporation

- *www.diabetespilot.com*

- *www.healthengage.com*

- *www.numedics.com/products/dppc/*
  Diabetes Partner PC software

CONTINUOUS SUBCUTANEOUS INSULIN INFUSION (CSII) RESOURCES

This list is not intended to be completely inclusive. It is intended to point educators and the people you educate to several beneficial and available resources.

Books for health care providers
- Bolderman, K.M. 2002. *Putting Your Patients on the Pump*. Alexandria, VA: American Diabetes Association.

Books for people with diabetes
- Kaplan-Mayer, G. 2003. *Insulin Pump Therapy Demystified: An Essential Guide for Pumping Insulin*. Westport, CT: Pub Group West.

- Walsh, J., R. Roberts. 2006. *Pumping Insulin: Everything You Need for Success on a Smart Insulin Pump*, 4th edition. San Diego: Torrey Pines Press.

- Wolpert, H., Editor. 2002. *Smart Pumping: A Practical Approach to Mastering the Insulin Pump*. Alexandria, VA: American Diabetes Association.

Consumer magazine publications for people with diabetes
- *Diabetes Forecast*. Alexandria, VA: American Diabetes Association. Monthly publication; often features CSII articles. The annual Resource Guide is an excellent tool for people considering or using CSII therapy. Website: *www.diabetes.org*; Phone: 800-806-7801

- *Diabetes Health*. Fairfax, CA. Monthly publication; contains Up & Pumping feature.
  Website: *www.DiabetesHealth.com*; Phone: 800-234-1218

- *Diabetes Self-Management*. New York, NY. Bi-monthly publication; often features insulin pump therapy articles. Phone: 800-234-0923

Useful articles
- Rice, D., K. Sweeney. 2006. Choosing and using an insulin pump infusion set. *Diabetes Self-Management* 23(November/December): 60–67.

- Scheiner, G. 2006. Go ahead, pick your pump: Which pump is right for you. *Diabetes Self-Management*, 23(November/December): 12–20.

Website

The website *www.diabetesnet.com* is an excellent online resource for information and products related to CSII. The following sections are especially helpful.

- Current insulin pumps:
  www.diabetesnet.com/diabetes_technology/insulinpumps.php

- Pump models and features:
  www.diabetesnet.com/diabetes_technology/insulin_pump_models.php

- Infusion sets:
  www.diabetesnet.com/diabetes_technology/infusion_sets.php

Blood Glucose–Lowering Medications

ORAL BLOOD GLUCOSE LOWERING MEDICATIONS

Category: Sulfonylureas*

Action: To stimulate insulin secretion in the pancreatic β-cells. (Can cause hypoglycemia.)

Generic Name	Trade Name	Common Dose	Usual Frequency
glimepiride	Amaryl	1, 2, 4 mg Max to 8 mg daily	One to two times daily
glipizide	Glucotrol Glucotrol XL (extended release)	2.5–5 mg Up to 40 mg daily; 20 mg with XL daily	One to two times daily (XL taken once daily)
glyburide	Diabeta Micronase Glynase PresTab	1.25–10 mg	One to two times daily

*Only second generation of sulfonylureas listed. First generation of these drugs are generally no longer in use.

Category: Meglinitinides

Action: To stimulate insulin secretion in the pancreatic β–cells. However, these have a shorter action time than sulfonylureas and are designed to be taken prior to meals to lower postprandial glucose. (Can cause hypoglycemia.)

Generic Name	Trade Name	Common Dose	Usual Frequency
repaglinide	Prandin	0.5–1.0 mg Up to 16 mg daily	Before meals, three times daily. Omit if meal not eaten.
nateglinide	Starlix	60–120 mg Up to 360 mg daily	Before meals, three times daily. Omit if meal not eaten.

Category: Biguanides

Action: Suppress glucose production in the liver and decrease insulin resistance. Increase glucose uptake by the muscles. (When taken as the only blood glucose–lowering agents and not in combination with another blood glucose–lowering agent, do not cause hypoglycemia.)

Generic Name	Trade Name	Common Dose	Usual Frequency
metformin	Glucophage Glucophage XR (extended release) Fortamet Riomet (liquid)	500–1,000 mg dose Up to 2,550 mg daily; max effective dose 2,000 mg daily	Two times a day. Slow titration suggested.

Category: Thiazolidinediones (TZDs)

Action: Decrease insulin resistance in adipose and muscle cells. (Taken as the only blood glucose–lowering agents and not in combination with another blood glucose–lowering agent, do not cause hypoglycemia.)

Generic Name	Trade Name	Common Dose	Usual Frequency
pioglitazone	Actos	15–45 mg	Once a day
rosiglitazone	Avandia	2–8 mg	Two times a day

Category: Alpha-Glucosidase inhibitors

Action: Decrease carbohydrate absorption in the gastrointestinal tract. (Taken as the only blood glucose–lowering agents and not in combination with another blood glucose–lowering agent, do not cause hypoglycemia.)

Generic Name	Trade Name	Common Dose	Usual Frequency
acarbose	Precose	Initiate at 25 mg and raise to max of 100 mg	With first bite of food at main meals
miglitol	Glyset	Initiate at 25 mg and raise to max of 100 mg	With first bite of food at main meals

Category: Dipeptidyl peptidase-4 inhibitors (DPP-4)

Action: Block the breakdown of glucagon-like peptide-1 (GLP-1) by blocking the effects of the enzyme dipeptidyl peptidase. This action helps to increase the synthesis and release of insulin from the pancreatic β–cells and decreases the release of glucagon from the pancreatic alpha cells in the presence of elevated blood glucose levels.

Generic Name	Trade Name	Common Dose	Usual Frequency
sitagliptin	Januvia	100 mg	Once a day

Combination meds

There is an increasing array of combinations of the above medications available for use in treating type 2 diabetes. They can be beneficial for some people by reducing the number of medications taken. However, it is more difficult to adjust each medication because the combinations are only available in certain dosage levels. Several of the combination medications available are:

- Actoplus Met—metformin + pioglitazone
- Avandamet—rosiglitazone + metformin
- Avandaryl—rosiglitazone + glimepiride
- Duetact—pioglitazone + glimepiride
- Glucovance—glyburide + metformin
- Janumet—metformin + sitagliptin
- Metaglip—glipizide + metformin

INJECTABLE BLOOD GLUCOSE LOWERING MEDICATIONS

Category: Incretin mimetics

Actions: Mimic the action of glucagon-like peptide (GLP-1) to increase insulin synthesis and secretion in the presence of elevated blood glucose levels, improve first-phase insulin response and reduce glucagon concentration when blood glucose is elevated, slow gastric emptying to slow the rise of blood glucose post meal and promote satiety (resulting in a lowered total calorie intake due to reduced hunger).

Generic Name	Trade Name	Common Dose	Usual Frequency
exenatide	BYETTA	5–10 µg in a pen that delivers the specified dose (either 5 or 10 µg)	Two times a day before morning and evening meals

Category: Amylin analog

Action: To help replace amylin, a hormone normally co-secreted with insulin from the pancreatic β-cells, in people with type 1 and insulin-requiring type 2 diabetes who have diminished amylin secretion. Pramlintide, the synthetic form of amylin, slows the rise of blood glucose after meals by slowing gastric emptying, suppressing glucagon secretion and promoting satiety (resulting in a lowered total calorie intake due to reduced hunger).

Generic Name	Trade Name	Common Dose	Usual Frequency
pramlintide acetate	SYMLIN	15 to 60 µg for type 1 Up to 120 µg for type 2	Taken before meals containing 30 g carbohydrate or 250 calories

Category: Insulin

Action: Lowers blood glucose levels by stimulating peripheral glucose uptake by the skeletal muscle and fat and by inhibiting hepatic glucose production. (Can cause hypoglycemia.)

Type of Insulin	Generic Name	Trade Name	Onset of Action	Peak of Action	Duration of Action
Rapid-acting	lispro	Humalog	5–15 minutes	1–2 hours	≤5 hours
	aspart	NovoLog			
	glulisine	Apridra			
Short-acting	regular, human	Humulin R Novolin R ReliOn	30–60 minutes	2–4 hours	6–10 hours
Intermediate	NPH, human	Humulin N Novolin N ReliOn	2–4 hours	4–10 hours	10–16 hours
Long-acting	glargine	Lantus	1–2 hours	Flat	20–24 hours
	detemir	Levemir			

Notes on insulin

1. Insulin action can vary from person to person. The onset, peak, and duration of action provided above are what is generally seen and reported in the literature.
2. Insulin is available in premixed combinations. These combinations are available as vials of insulin or insulin pens. The combinations available today are generally combinations of NPH and regular insulin or a combination of insulin analogs. Common combinations are 70/30, 75/25, and 50/50 with the longer-acting component providing the larger amount.
3. Insulin is generally given in combinations, either through the use of two insulins injected individually, i.e., a long-acting insulin once or twice a day with a rapid-acting insulin at mealtimes, or a premixed insulin provided twice a day. The action curves for common combinations of insulin are provided in chapter 12.

Several references were utilized to develop these tables (Childs and Kruger 2005; Steil 2006).

Sample Record Keeping for Basic and Advanced Carbohydrate Counting

Carbohydrate Counting and Blood Glucose Results Record

Day/Date: _____

Time/Meal	Diabetes Medicines		Food		carb count (choices/grams)	Blood Glucose Results							
	type	amount	type	amount		Fasting/ Before Break-fast	After Break-fast	Before Lunch	After Lunch	Before Dinner	After Dinner	Before Bed	Other

Notes about day:

Insulin Pump Therapy Record

Name: _____ Insulin Pump: _____ Insulin: _____

Day/Date: _____ Glucose Meter: _____

Target Blood Glucose: _____ mg/dl Correction Factor: _____ mg/dl Duration of Insulin Action: _____ hours

Basal rate	units/hour
12:00 midnight	

Basal Pattern: _____ Basal total: _____ u/day

Insulin: Carbohydrate Ratio: 1 unit: _____ g carbohydrate AND/OR Custom Boluses

1 unit: _____ g carbohydrate for brkfst (Custom bolus): 1 unit: _____ g carb, _____ % immed, _____ % over _____ h

1 unit: _____ g carbohydrate for lunch (Custom bolus): 1 unit: _____ g carb, _____ % immed, _____ % over _____ h

1 unit: _____ g carbohydrate for dinner (Custom bolus): 1 unit: _____ g carb, _____ % immed, _____ % over _____ h

Time	12A	1A	2A	3A	4A	5A	6A	7A	8A	9A	10A	11A	12P	1P	2P	3P	4P	5P	6P	7P	8P	9P	10P	11P
Basal rate u/h																								
Glucose mg/dl																								
Carbohydrate grams																								
Food bolus (u)																								
Correction bolus (u)																								
Set change																								

Comments/Assessment: _____

Plan: _____ continue current regimen OR _____ change regimen to: _____

Flowsheet for Carbohydrate Counting and MDI Therapy—5 Days

My insulin: carb ratio: 1 unit _____ gm carb.

My correction factor: 1 unit ↓bg _____ mg/dl

I correct a high blood glucose to a target of: _____ mg/dl

Day/Date	12A	6A	7A	8A	9A	10A	11A	12N	1P	2P	3P	4P	5P	6P	7P	8P	9P	10P	11P
BG																			
Carb grams																			
Food bolus																			
Corr. bolus																			
Total Bolus																			

Day/Date	12A	6A	7A	8A	9A	10A	11A	12N	1P	2P	3P	4P	5P	6P	7P	8P	9P	10P	11P
BG																			
Carb grams																			
Food bolus																			
Corr. bolus																			
Total Bolus																			

Day/Date	12A		6A	7A	8A	9A	10A	11A	12N	1P	2P	3P	4P	5P	6P	7P	8P	9P	10P	11P
BG																				
Carb grams																				
Food bolus																				
Corr. bolus																				
Total Bolus																				

Day/Date	12A		6A	7A	8A	9A	10A	11A	12N	1P	2P	3P	4P	5P	6P	7P	8P	9P	10P	11P
BG																				
Carb grams																				
Food bolus																				
Corr. bolus																				
Total Bolus																				

Day/Date	12A		6A	7A	8A	9A	10A	11A	12N	1P	2P	3P	4P	5P	6P	7P	8P	9P	10P	11P
BG																				
Carb grams																				
Food bolus																				
Corr. bolus																				
Total Bolus																				

Flowsheet for Carbohydrate Counting and Insulin Pump Therapy—4 Days

	Begin time	Units/hr
Rate 1	12 AM	
Rate 2		
Rate 3		
Rate 4		
Rate 5		

My insulin: carb ratio: 1 unit _____ gm carb.
My correction factor: 1 unit ↓bg _____ mg/dl
I correct a high blood glucose to a target of: _____ mg/dl

Day/Date	12A	6A	7A	8A	9A	10A	11A	12N	1P	2P	3P	4P	5P	6P	7P	8P	9P	10P	11P
BG																			
Carb grams																			
Food bolus																			
Corr. bolus																			
Insulin-on-board																			
Total Bolus																			
Temp basal																			
Set Change? (note time of change with X)																			

Day/Date	12A	6A	7A	8A	9A	10A	11A	12N	1P	2P	3P	4P	5P	6P	7P	8P	9P	10P	11P
BG																			
Carb grams																			
Food bolus																			
Corr. bolus																			
Insulin-on-board																			
Total Bolus																			
Temp basal																			
Set Change? (note time of change with X)																			

Day/Date	12A		6A	7A	8A	9A	10A	11A	12N	1P	2P	3P	4P	5P	6P	7P	8P	9P	10P	11P
BG																				
Carb grams																				
Food bolus																				
Corr. bolus																				
Insulin-on-board																				
Total Bolus																				
Temp basal																				
Set Change? (note time of change with X)																				

Day/Date	12A		6A	7A	8A	9A	10A	11A	12N	1P	2P	3P	4P	5P	6P	7P	8P	9P	10P	11P
BG																				
Carb grams																				
Food bolus																				
Corr. bolus																				
Insulin-on-board																				
Total Bolus																				
Temp basal																				
Set Change? (note time of change with X)																				

Reference List

Reference List

Ahern, J.A., P.M. Gatcomb, N.A. Held, W.A. Petit, W.V. Tamborlane. 1993. Exaggerated hyperglycemia after a pizza meal in well-controlled diabetes. *Diabetes Care* 16:578–580.

American Diabetes Association. 2003. Flying with diabetes. *Clinical Diabetes* 21:86.

———. 2005. Care of children and adolescents with type 1 diabetes. *Diabetes Care* 28:186–212.

———. 2008a. Clinical practice recommendations. *Diabetes Care* 31:S1–S110.

———. 2008b. Nutrition recommendations and interventions for diabetes. *Diabetes Care* 29:2149–2157.

American Diabetes Association, American Dietetic Association. 2008. *Choose your foods: Exchange lists for diabetes.* Alexandria, VA: American Diabetes Association, Chicago: American Dietetic Association.

Anderson, E.J., M. Richardson, G. Castle, S. Cercone, L. Delahanty, R. Lyon, D. Mueller, L. Snetselaar. 1993. Nutrition interventions for intensive therapy in the Diabetes Control and Complications Trial. *J Am Diet Assoc* 93:768–772.

Aronoff, S.L., K. Berkowitz, B. Shreiner, L. Want. 2004. Glucose metabolism and regulation: beyond insulin and glucagon. *Diabetes Spectrum* 17:183–190.

Balkau, B., M. Shipley, R.J. Jarrett, K. Pyorala, M. Pyorala, et al. 1998. High blood glucose concentration is a risk factor for mortality in middle-aged non-diabetic men: 20-year follow-up in the Whitehall Study, the Paris Prospective Study, and the Helsinki Policeman Study. *Diabetes Care* 21:360–367.

Bode, B., ed. 2004. *Medical management of type 1 diabetes*, 4th ed. Alexandria, VA: American Diabetes Association.

Bolderman, K.M. 2002. *Putting your patients on the pump.* Alexandria, VA: American Diabetes Association.

Bowman, S.A., B.T. Vinyard. 2004. Fast food consumption of U.S. adults: Impact on energy and nutrient intakes and overweight status. *J Am Coll Nutr* 23:163–168.

Braithwaite, S.S. 2005. Case study: Five steps to freedom: Dose titration for type 2 diabetes using basal-prandial correction insulin therapy. *Clinical Diabetes* 23:39–43.

Brand-Miller, J., S. Hayne, P. Petocz, S. Colagiuri. 2003. Low-glycemic index diets in the management of diabetes: A meta-analysis of randomized controlled trials. *Diabetes Care* 26:2261–2267.

Burdick, J., H.P. Chase, R.H. Slover, K. Knievel, L. Scrimgeour, et al. 2004. Missed insulin meal boluses and elevated hemoglobin A1C levels in children receiving insulin pump therapy. *Pediatrics* 113: 221–224.

BYETTA. 2007. [Package insert]. San Diego, CA: Amylin Pharmaceuticals, Inc. http://pi.lilly.com/us/byetta-pi.pdf (accessed March 3, 2008).

Case, A., R.L. Reid. 1998. Effects of the menstrual cycle on medical disorders. *Arch Intern Med* 158:1405–1412.

Ceriello, A. 2005. Postprandial hyperglycemia and diabetes: Is it time to treat? *Diabetes* 54:1–7.

Ceriello, A., J. Davidson, M. Hanefeld, L. Leiter, L. Monnier, et al. 2006. Postprandial hyperglycemia and cardiovascular complications of diabetes: An update. *Nutrition, Metabolism & Cardiovascular Disease* 16:453–456.

Chase, H.P., S.Z. Saib, T. MacKenzie, M.M. Hansen, S.K. Garg. 2002. Postprandial glucose excursions following four methods of bolus insulin administration in subjects with type 1 diabetes. *Diabetic Medicine* 19:317–21.

Childs, B.P., D. Kruger. 2005. Treatment strategies for type 1 diabetes. In *Complete nurse's guide to diabetes care,* ed. Childs, B.P., M. Cypress, G. Spollett, 37. Alexandria, VA: American Diabetes Association.

Colberg, S. 2001. *The diabetic athlete.* Champaign, IL: Human Kinetics.

Coutinho, M., H.C. Gerstein, Y. Wang, S. Yusuf. 1999. The relationship between glucose and incident cardiovascular events: A metaregression analysis of published data from 20 studies of 95,783 individuals followed for 12.4 years. *Diabetes Care* 22:233–240.

DAFNE Study Group. 2002. Training in flexible, intensive insulin management to enable dietary freedom in people with type 1 diabetes: Dose adjustment for normal eating (DAFNE) randomized controlled trial. *Brit Med J* 325:746–752.

Davidson, P.C., H.R. Hebblewhite, B.W. Bode, P.L. Richardson, R.D. Steed, et al. 2003. Statistical estimates for CSII parameters: carbohydrate-to-insulin ratio (CIR); correction factor (CF); and basal insulin. *Diabetes Technol Ther* 5:A28.

Davidson, P.C., H.R. Hebblewhite, B.W. Bode, R.D. Steed, N.S. Welch, et al. 2003. Statistically based CSII parameters: correction factor, CF (1700 rule), carbohydrate-to-insulin ratio, CIR (2.8 rule), and basal-to-total ratio. *Diabetes Technol Ther* 3:237.

Davidson, P.C., R.D. Steed, B.W. Bode. 2003. Deductive framework to aid in understanding CSII parameters: Carbohydrate-to-insulin ratio (CIR) and correction factor (CF). *Diabetes* 52:S443.

de Vegt, F., J.M. Dekker, H.G. Ruhe, C.D.A. Stehouwer, G.B.L.M. Nijpels, et al. 1999. Hyperglycaemia is associated with all-cause and cardiovascular mortality in the Hoorn population: The Hoorn Study. *Diabetologia* 42:926–931.

The DECODE Study Group, the European Diabetes Epidemiology Group. 1999. Glucose tolerance and mortality: Comparison of WHO and American Diabetes Association diagnostic criteria. *Lancet* 354:617–621.

Diabetes Control and Complications Trial Research Group. 1993. The effect of intensive treatment of diabetes on the development and progression of long-term complications in insulin-dependent diabetes mellitus. *N Engl J Med* 329:977–986.

———. 1997. Weight gain associated with intensive therapy in the Diabetes Control and Complications Trial. *Diabetes Care* 11:67–73.

Donahue, R.P., R.D. Abbot, D.M. Reed, K. Yano. 1987. Postchallenge glucose concentration and coronary heart disease in men of Japanese ancestry: Honolulu Heart Program. *Diabetes* 36:689–692.

Dougherty, P., J.G. Pastors. 2007. Menopause: What to expect, how to cope. *Diabetes Self-Management* 24:85.

Evert, A. 2006. Pump corner: What "rule" do you use? *Newsflash* (Diabetes Care and Education Practice Group of the American Dietetic Association) 27:29.

Feigenbaum, K. 2006. Treating gastroparesis. *Diabetes Self-Management* 23:24–28.

Franz, M.J. 2000. Protein controversies in diabetes. *Diabetes Spectrum* 13:132.

Franz, M.J. 2002. Nutrition, physical activity, and diabetes. In *Handbook of exercise in diabetes*, ed. Ruderman, N., J.T. Devlin, S.H. Schneider, A. Kriska, 337. Alexandra, VA: American Diabetes Association.

Franz, M.J., J.P. Bantle, C.A. Beebe, J.D. Brunzell, J.L. Chiasson, et al. 2002. Evidence-based nutrition principles and recommendations for the treatment and prevention of diabetes and related complications. *Diabetes Care* 25:148–198.

Gannon, M.C., J.A. Nuttall, G. Damberg, V. Gupta, F.Q. Nuttall. 2001. Effect of protein ingestion on the glucose appearance rate in people with type 2 diabetes. *J Clin Endocrinol Metab* 86:1040–1047.

Garg, S., H. Zisser, S. Schwartz, T. Bailey, R. Kaplan, et al. 2006. Improvement in glycemic excursions with a transcutaneous, real-time continuous sensor: A randomized controlled trial. *Diabetes Care* 29:44–50.

Hinnen, D., D. Guthrie, B. Childs, R.A. Guthrie. 2003. Pattern management of blood glucose. In *A core curriculum for diabetes education, diabetes management therapies*, 5th ed., ed. Franz, M.J. Chicago: American Association of Diabetes Educators.

Hinnen, D., R.A. Guthrie. 2005. Self-management practices. In *Complete nurse's guide to diabetes care*, ed. Childs, B.P., M. Cypress, G. Spollett, 64. Alexandria, VA: American Diabetes Association.

Hirsch, I.B. 2005. Insulin analogues. *N Engl J Med* 352:174–183.

Hirsch, I.B., R.F. Hirsch. 2001. View 2: Sliding scale or sliding scare: It's all sliding nonsense. *Diabetes Spectrum* 14:79–81.

Homko, C.J. 2005. Women and diabetes. In *Complete nurse's guide to diabetes care*, ed. Childs, B.P., M. Cypress, G. Spollett, 279. Alexandria, VA: American Diabetes Association.

Hoogwerf, B.J. 2006. Exenatide and pramlintide: New glucose-lowering agents for treating diabetes mellitus. *Cleveland Clinic Journal of Medicine* 73:477–484.

Howey, D.C., R.R. Bowsher, R.L. Brunelle, J.R. Wentworth. 1994. [Lys(B28), Pro(B29)]-human insulin: A rapidly absorbed analogue of human insulin. *Diabetes* 43:396–402.

Institute of Medicine. 2002. *Dietary reference intakes: Energy, carbohydrate, fiber, fat, fatty acids, cholesterol, protein and amino acids*. Washington, D.C.: National Academies Press.

Jones, S.M., J.L. Quarry, M. Caldwell-McMillan, D. Mauger, R. Gabbay. 2005. Optimal insulin pump dosing and postprandial glycemia following a pizza meal using the continuous glucose monitoring system. *Diabetes Technology & Therapeutics* 7:233–240.

Karl, D.M. 2006. Learning to use pramlintide. *Practical Diabetology* March, 5–8.

Keith, K., D. Nicholson, D. Rogers. 2004. Accuracy and precision of low-dose administration using syringes, pens, and a pump. *Clinical Pediatrics* 43:69–74.

King, A.B., D.U. Armstrong. 2007. A prospective evaluation of insulin dosing recommendations in patients with type 1 diabetes at near normal glucose control: Bolus dosing. *Journal of Diabetes Science and Technology* 1:42–46.

Kruger, D. 2006. Symlin and Byetta: Two new antihyperglycemic medications. *Practical Diabetology* March, 9–12.

Kruger, D.F., M.A. Gloster. 2004. Pramlintide for the treatment of insulin-requiring diabetes mellitus: Rationale and review of clinical data. *Drugs* 64:1419–1432.

Levetan, C., L.L. Want, C. Weyer, S.A. Strobel, J. Crean, et al. 2003. Impact of pramlintide on glucose fluctuations and postprandial glucose, glucagon, and triglyceride excursions among patients with type 1 diabetes intensively treated with insulin pumps. *Diabetes Care* 26:1–8.

Lowe, L.P., K. Liu, P. Greenland, B.E. Metzger, A.R. Dyer, et al. 1997. Diabetes, asymptomatic hyperglycemia, and 22-year mortality in black and white men: The Chicago Heart Association Detection Project in Industry study. *Diabetes Care* 20:163–169.

Lustman, P.J., R.J. Anderson, K.E. Freedland, M. de Groot, R.M. Carney, et al. 2000. Depression and poor glycemic control: A meta-analytic review of the literature. *Diabetes Care* 23:934–942.

Maia, F.F., L.R. Araujo. 2007. Efficacy of continuous glucose monitoring system (CGMS) to detect postprandial hyperglycemia and unrecognized hypoglycemia in type 1 diabetes patients. *Diabetes Res Clin Pract* 75:30–34.

McCulloch, D.K., R.D. Mitchell, J. Mabler, R.B. Tatttersall. 1993. Influence of imaginative teaching of diet on compliance and metabolic control in insulin dependent diabetes. *Brit J Med* 287:1858–1862.

Melki, V., F. Ayon, M. Fernandez, H. Hanaire-Broutin. Value and limitations of the continuous glucose monitoring system in the management of type 1 diabetes. *Diabetes Metab* 32:123–129.

Moberg, E., M. Kollind, P.E. Lins, U. Adamson. 1995. Day-to-day variation of insulin sensitivity in patients with type 1 diabetes: Role of gender and menstrual cycle. *Diabet Med* 12:224–228.

Monnier, L., C. Colette. 2006. Contributions of fasting and postprandial glucose to hemoglobin A1c. *Endocr Pract* 12(Suppl 1):42–46.

Mudaliar, S., R.A. Lindberg, M. Joyce, P. Beerdsen, P. Strange, et al. 1999. Insulin aspart (B28 Asp-insulin): A fast-acting analog of human insulin: Absorption kinetics and action profile compared with regular human insulin in healthy nondiabetic subjects. *Diabetes Care* 22:1501–1506.

Mullooly, C.A. 2006. Physical activity. In *The art and science of diabetes self-management education*, ed. Mensing, C., M. Cypres, C. Halstenson, S. McLaughlin, E.A. Walker, 307–308. Chicago: American Association of Diabetes Educators.

National Restaurant Association. 2008. *2008 restaurant industry forecast.* Washington, DC; National Restaurant Association.

Nauck, M.A., M.M. Heimesaat, C. Orskov, J.J. Holst, R. Ebert, et al. 1993. Preserved incretin activity of glucagon-like-peptide 1 (7-36 amide) but not of synthetic human gastric inhibitory polypeptide in patients with type-2 diabetes mellitus. *J Clin Invest* 91:301–307.

Nowak, T.V., C.P. Johnson, J.H. Kalbfleisch, A.M. Roza, C.M. Wood, et al. 1995. Highly variable gastric emptying in patients with insulin dependent diabetes mellitus. *Gut* 37:23–29.

Parkin, C., N. Brooks. 2002. Is postprandial glucose control important? Is it practical in primary care settings? *Clinical Diabetes* 20:71–76.

Pastors, J.G., H. Warshaw, A. Daly, M. Franz, K. Kulkarni. 2002. The evidence for the effectiveness of medical nutrition therapy in diabetes management. *Diabetes Care* 25:608–613.

Pastors, J.G., M. Arnold, A. Daly, M. Franz, H. Warshaw. 2003. *Diabetes nutrition Q & A for health professionals*. Alexandria, VA: American Diabetes Association.

Pastors, J.G., M.J. Franz, H. Warshaw, A. Daly, M.S. Arnold. 2003. How effective is medical nutrition therapy in diabetes care? *J Am Diet Assoc* 103:827–831.

Pereira, M.A., A.I. Kartashov, C.B. Ebbeling, L. Van Horn, M.L. Slattery, D.R. Jacobs Jr., D.S. Ludwig. 2005. Fast-food habits, weight gain, and insulin resistance (the CARDIA study): 15-year prospective analysis. *Lancet* 365:36–42.

Perley, M.J., D.M. Kipnis. 1967. Plasma insulin responses to oral and intravenous glucose studies in normal and diabetic subjects. *J Clin Invest* 46:1954–1962.

Peters, A.L., M.B. Davidson. 1993. Protein and fat effects on glucose responses and insulin requirements in subjects with insulin-dependent diabetes mellitus. *Am J Clin Nutrition* 58:555–560.

Pickup, J., H. Kenn. 2002. Continuous subcutaneous insulin infusion at 25 years: Evidence base for the expanding use of insulin pump therapy in type 1 diabetes. *Diabetes Care*; 25:593–598.

Polonsky, W.H., R.A. Jackson. 2004. What's so tough about taking insulin? Addressing the problem of psychological insulin resistance in type 2 diabetes. *Clinical Diabetes* 22:147–150.

Rassam, A.G., R.M. Zeise, M.R. Burge, D.S. Schade. 1999. Optimal administration of lispro insulin in hyperglycemic type 1 diabetes. *Diabetes Care* 22:133–136.

Riddle, M.C., D.J. Drucker. 2006. Emerging therapies mimicking the effects of amylin and glucagon-like peptide 1. *Diabetes Care* 29:435–449.

Rosenstock, J., S.L. Schwartz, C.M. Clark, G.D. Park, D.W. Donley, et al. 2001. Basal insulin therapy in type 2 diabetes: 28-week comparison of insulin glargine (HOE 901) and NPH insulin. *Diabetes Care* 24:631–636.

Rosetti, P., S. Pampanelli, C. Fanelli, F. Porcellati, E. Costa, et al. 2003. Intensive replacement of basal insulin in patients with type 1 diabetes given rapid-acting insulin analog at mealtime: A 3-month comparison between administration of NPH insulin four times daily and glargine insulin at dinner or bedtime. *Diabetes Care* 26:1490–1496.

Schade, D.S., V. Valentine. 2006. Are insulin pumps underutilized in type 1 diabetes? No. *Diabetes Care* 29:1443–1444.

Scheiner, G. 2006. The great blood glucose balancing act. *Diabetes Self-Management* 23:51.

Schwide-Slavin, C. 2003. Case study: A patient with type 1 diabetes who transitions to insulin pump therapy by working with an advanced practice dietitian. *Diabetes Spectrum* 16:37–40.

Sheard, N., N. Clark, J.C. Brand-Miller, M.J. Franz, F.X. Pi-Sunyer, E. Mayer-Davis, K. Kulkarni, P. Geil. 2004. Dietary carbohydrate (amount and type) in the prevention and management of diabetes: A statement by the American Diabetes Association. *Diabetes Care* 27:2266–2271.

Skovlund, S.E., M. Peyrot (on behalf of the DAWN International Advisory Panel). 2005. The Diabetes Attitudes, Wishes, and Needs (DAWN) program: A new approach to improving outcomes of diabetes care. *Diabetes Spectrum* 18:136–142.

Skyler, J.S. 2004. Insulin treatment. In *Therapy for diabetes mellitus and related disorders*, 4th ed., ed. Lebovitz, H.E., 207–223. Alexandria, VA: American Diabetes Association.

Steil, C.F. 2006. Pharmacologic therapies for glucose management. In *The art and science of diabetes self-nanagement education*, ed. Mensing, C., M. Cypress, C. Halstenson, S. McLaughlin, E.A. Walker, 321–355. Chicago: American Association of Diabetes Educators.

SYMLIN. 2007. [Package insert]. San Diego, CA: Amylin Pharmaceuticals, Inc. http://symlin.com/pdf/symlin-pi-combined.pdf (accessed March 3, 2008).

Temelkova-Kurktschiev, T.S., C. Koehler, E. Henkel, W. Leonhardt, K. Fuecker, M. Hanefeld. 2000. Postchallenge plasma glucose and glycemic spikes are more strongly associated with atherosclerosis than fasting glucose or HbA1c level. *Diabetes Care* 23:1830–1834.

U.K. Prospective Diabetes Study Group. 1998. Intensive blood-glucose control with sulphonylureas or insulin compared with conventional treatment and risk of complications in patients with type 2 diabetes (UKPDS 33). *Lancet* 352:837–853.

U.S. Department of Health and Human Services and U.S. Department of Agriculture. 2005. Adequate nutrients within calorie needs. In *Dietary guidelines for Americans 2005*. Washington, D.C.: U.S. Department of Health and Human Services and U.S. Department of Agriculture. http://www.healthierus.gov/dietaryguidelines (accessed April 9, 2008).

U.S. Food and Drug Administration. 2004. *How to understand and use a food label*. Washington, D.C.: U.S. Food and Drug Administration. http://www.cfsan.fda.gov/~acrobat/foodlab.pdf (accessed April 9, 2008).

192 Practical Carbohydrate Counting

Wallum, B.J., S.E. Kahn, D.K. McCulloch, D. Porte. 1992. Insulin secretion in the normal and diabetic human. In *International textbook of diabetes mellitus*, ed. Alberti, K.G.M.M., R.A. DeFronzo, H. Keen, P. Zimmer, 285–301. Chichester, U.K.: John Wiley and Sons.

Walsh, J., R. Roberts. 2006. *Pumping insulin: Everything you need for success on a smart insulin pump*, 4th ed. San Diego, CA: Torrey Pines Press.

Walsh, J., R. Roberts, C. Varma, T. Bailey. 2003. Which insulin to use and how to start. In *Using insulin*. San Diego, CA: Torrey Pines Press.

Want, L.L., R. Ratner. 2006. Pramlintide: A new tool in diabetes management. *Current Diabetes Reports* 6:344–349.

Warshaw, H.S. 2005. Rapid-acting insulin: Action curve update with practical tips. *On the Cutting Edge* 26:12–15.

Warshaw, H.S. 2005. Rapid-acting insulin: Timing it just right. *Diabetes Self-Management* 22:20–25.

Warshaw, H.S., M. Powers. 1999. A search for answers about foods with polyols (sugar alcohols). *Diabetes Educator* 25:307–321.

Weyer, C., D.G. Maggs, A.A. Young, O.G. Kolterman. 2001. Amylin replacement with pramlintide as an adjunct to insulin therapy in type 1 and type 2 diabetes mellitus: A physiological approach toward improved metabolic control. *Curr Pharm Des* 7:1353–1373.

Wolpert, H., ed. 2002. *Smart pumping: A practical approach to mastering the insulin pump*. Alexandria, VA: American Diabetes Association.

Index

Index

Note: Page numbers followed by a t refer to tables. Page numbers followed by an f refer to figures.

physical activity, 135t
pump therapy, 70, 72–79, 81–83, 160
vacation, 139, 141

K

Ketones, 91t–92t, 94t, 107, 134, 137–139
Ketosis, 134, 137–139
King, Allen B., 61

L

Lifestyle changes, 40, 43, 59, 63, 71, 73, 86, 133, 139
Lipids, 1, 2t
Lipoprotein levels, 1, 2t
Liver, 122

M

Medical Nutrition Therapy (MNT). *See* Nutrition
Menopause, 73, 142
Menses, 53, 57, 71, 86, 91t, 94t–95t, 97, 142
Multiple daily injections (MDI) regimen
carbohydrate counting and, 5–6, 51–53, 55, 178–179
hypoglycemia, 24, 63
and insulin therapy, 65, 71, 147–148
macronutrients effect on, 123
pharmacological therapy, 75, 154
postprandial capillary plasma glucose, 38
sick day management, 138–139

N

NASCO, 37
Nutrition. *See also* Carbohydrate counting; Carbohydrate(s)
caloric intake, 7, 20–21, 29, 139
carbohydrate counting education, 12
children, 29, 68
exchanges/choices, 27, 31–32
fats, dietary, 7, 17–19, 29, 67, 75, 89t, 93t, 121–122, 141
fiber, dietary, 19, 67, 125, 141
food database, personal, 159t
food diary, 57, 96t
food groups, 26–27
food habits, case studies, 39–40, 42–43, 45–46, 108, 112–113
goals, 28–29
individual needs, 1, 68
meal planning, 25t, 27
case studies, 40, 43, 46
pattern management, 86–87
polyols (sugar alcohols), 130–131
portion control, 31–37, 157–160
preferences, 1
pregnancy, 29, 68
protein, 7, 17–19, 29, 35, 75, 89t, 93t, 121–122
restaurants, portion control tips for eating at, 36, 128–130, 166
serving sizes, 26–27
sucrose, dietary, 27–28, 131
"sugars", 32–33
vitamins and minerals, 19–20, 141
Nutrition Counseling and Education Services, 37
Nutrition Facts panel, 13, 26, 28, 31–37, 131–132, 157–160

Other Titles From The
American Diabetes Association

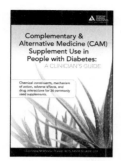
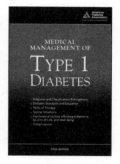
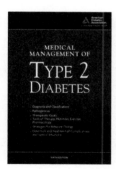
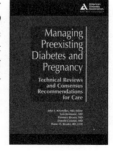